A
SIMPLE
PLAN

A SIMPLE PLAN

*Alternative Medicine
Made Very Easy*

Colleen C. Badell, Ph.D.

Turning Point Press
Napa, California

Turning Point Press
P.O. Box 4111
Napa, California 94558–0411

Printed in the United States of America

For more information, visit www.health-advocate.com

Interior typesetting by Desktop Miracles
Index by Linzer Indexing Services
Cartoons rendered by Erin Leong

Library of Congress Control Number 2004098447
ISBN 0-9761129-0-6

CIP data available

To my father who often said,
what you keep to yourself, you lose;
what you give away, you keep forever.

—ATTRIBUTED TO FRANCIS QUARLES, 1632

A Short History of Medicine

Doctor, "I have an earache."

2000 B.C. "Here, eat this root."

1000 B.C. "That root is heathen, say this prayer."

1850 A.D. "That prayer is superstition, drink this potion."

1940 A.D. "That potion is snake oil, swallow this pill."

1985 A.D. "That pill is ineffective, take this antibiotic."

2000 A.D. "That antibiotic is artificial, eat this root."

—THE INTERNET

Contents

Preface   9

Acknowledgments   13

INTRODUCTION Why Another Guide?   15

CHAPTER 1   Alternative Versus Conventional Medicine   23

CHAPTER 2   How to Choose & Use an Alternative
                Medicine Practitioner   37

CHAPTER 3   How to Choose & Use a Psychotherapist   53

CHAPTER 4   How to Choose & Use an Alternative
                Medicine Remedy   71

CHAPTER 5   Six Steps to Using Alternative Medicine   89

                STEP ONE   Assess Your Lifestyle   95

                STEP TWO   Balance Your Space   125

                STEP THREE Balance Your Energy   136

                STEP FOUR   Balance Your Mind   150

                STEP FIVE   Balance Your Body   176

                STEP SIX   Prevent Future Imbalance   186

CHAPTER 6   Use Alternative Medicine to Survive Surgery   193

CHAPTER 7   Approach Death & Dying with a New View   205

CHAPTER 8   Conclusion   219

APPENDIX A Professional Associations & Organizations   225

APPENDIX B Internet Resources   237

APPENDIX C Six-Step Workbook   241

Bibliography   251

Index   255

PREFACE

As a health strategist and consumer advocate, I am dedicated to helping people get the most from their health care including the safe, responsible, and effective use of alternative medicine. My initial interest in integrating conventional medicine with alternative medicine began on a late 1960s college campus where a renewed interest in Eastern ideology and philosophy emerged. Experimentation with alternative lifestyles led to a new approach to disease prevention and health maintenance through the use of alternative methodologies.

Most people develop a commitment to their health only after a catastrophic event forces them to do so, but this wasn't true for me. I always had a keen interest in all aspects of my health—physical, mental, and spiritual—which was further ignited when I discovered alternative medicine. As a nonconformist, questioning the status quo of conventional medicine came naturally to me, particularly when it was inadequate in addressing my needs. The concept of non-invasive, natural methods of treatment, based on medicine thousands of years old that was effective without being harmful, appealed to my pragmatic and health-conscious nature.

I adopted a proactive attitude toward my health care, trying different alternative methods over the years and learning to follow my own counsel. Among the first practices I used were biological medicine, nutritional supplementation, meditation, yoga, and modified vegetarianism. Much to my surprise, I found that several Eastern wisdom traditions closely matched my own philosophy of life. I did all this while maintaining a conventional business career in an environment that was not altogether sympathetic to my activities.

In fact, when I began using alternative medicine, there was little understanding or tolerance for it at all. Tofu and mantra jokes were extremely popular. Those of us who used it were often described as "a little left of magnetic north," and I learned to keep my practices to myself. Those of us who persevered during these times did so for the sole reason that we believed in alternative medicine and knew it worked through sometimes frustrating trial and error. It was simply worth the occasional taunts and cross-examinations.

Through many years of good health with minor bouts of illness, I discovered alternative methods that were repeatedly and sometimes remarkably effective. I learned the importance of discernment in choosing not only the right alternative medicine but the right alternative practitioner and the value of pursuing the underlying causes of illness rather than the immediate resolution of symptoms. Alternative medicine was all about what you did for yourself rather than what others did for you. When I did experience a serious health crisis many years later, I was able to resolve it completely through an integrated approach to health, contrary to the predictions of my doctors.

Like anyone who has used alternative medicine for a long time, I have experienced both the pleasures and perils of using this medicine. I know how confusing it can be and how difficult it is to get reliable, unbiased information. Alternative medicine may be inaccessible to consumers for many reasons:

- an absence of support from the conventional medical establishment

- a confusing number of alternative practices from which to choose

- the conflicting approaches of many alternative practices

- the time and expense needed to investigate alternative treatment options

- a lack of scientific documentation on many alternative therapies

- a fear of harm or exploitation by incompetent or fraudulent alternative practitioners

I don't advocate or support any particular alternative medicine practice. I do advocate an activist and informed approach to health care, conventional or alternative. The alternative practices briefly discussed in the guide are offered merely as examples to illustrate the six-step plan and to provide a framework for using alternative medicine. They do not constitute all the alternative practices that are available. My intent is not to choose a practice for you but to provide you with the power to make your own informed choices and to raise issues that may be helpful in your search for healing.

The purpose of the guide is also not to document the effectiveness of alternative medicine through scientific study. General reference to science is made in order to confirm the effectiveness of a treatment or to emphasize the importance of a particular health issue. There are many good books on alternative medicine and science, many of which are recommended throughout the guide.

Not only does the guide encourage better and more responsible consumerism of alternative medicine, but it also presents a broader view of wellness and illness, which hopefully serves to elevate the stakes in health care. In doing so, a better understanding of alternative medicine is possible, fostering its use and acceptance in mainstream society. It also presents this view in clear and simple terms, so instead of spending all your time trying to figure out what to do, you can focus more on actually doing.

The information contained in the guide has helped me and others make smart health care choices, representing the culmination of more than three decades of successes and failures in an effort to find an approach to medicine that works. But it is only useful to the extent that you can adapt it to suit your own individual needs and requirements.

As the sixth-century Taoist philosopher Lao Tzu said, "The journey of a thousand miles begins with one step." Only if you decide the task is worth the effort will the information in this guide be of use to you. It is offered as a source of clarity in the maze of confusion—in a spirit of cooperation rather than competition.

ACKNOWLEDGMENTS

This guide is a tribute to the pioneering people who discussed and supported alternative medicine at a time when it was neither popular nor profitable, setting an example for us all. I am grateful to the many practitioners and teachers who have shared their knowledge and wisdom with me over the decades.

My thanks to former Harper Collins editor Carolyn Pinkus for setting me on the right path. Friends Bill Knowles, David Walker, and Kathy vanderVennet, and Copperfield Books' Christine Jawski provided helpful suggestions and proofing skills along the way, as did Harv Chapman along with his formidable artistic talents. English Professor Don Gray gave very generously of his time, and computer gurus Mike Eshelman and Steve Adams went the extra mile to keep me up and running, hardware and software-wise.

Many of the ideas presented in this guide about life, death, and healing are based on universal laws of nature that have been experienced and written about by many people throughout the history of time. No one has a copyright on this wisdom; it belongs to all of us. This guide is based on my personal philosophy and experiences. I have made every effort to document sources of information other than my own. If I have failed to give proper credit where credit is due, the fault is entirely mine.

INTRODUCTION

WHY ANOTHER GUIDE?

Why do we need another guide to alternative medicine when there are already dozens of them on the market? Therein lies the problem. Most of the guides to alternative medicine offer the same thing: encyclopedic lists of practices, techniques, therapies, remedies, and health conditions. They work well if you want to know all of the alternative practices that exist in the universe or all of the alternative treatments recommended for a particular health condition. They do not work well if you do not know what your condition is or which alternative practice to use. These guides almost never address how to find a good practitioner.

This guide attempts to fill that gap and do so with the type of straight talk you are not likely to hear from most health professionals. It simplifies the complex, organizing alternative medicine in such a way that makes it easier to use with consideration for your own individual needs. It provides:

- a broader view of healing—redefining what it means and your role in the process

- a practical context for using alternative medicine safely and effectively

- specific guidelines for making wise alternative choices and avoiding the pitfalls of making poor ones

- a simplified presentation of systems, modalities, and methods of alternative medicine

- a manageable number of resources and tools designed to make alternative medicine more accessible and usable

Consumer Advocate Viewpoint

This guide attempts to provide uncensored information in the most straightforward terms about how to choose and use alternative medicine. This is *health care with an attitude*, which is defined as the only way to survive a system of medicine—and alternative medicine is fast becoming part of that system—that has become more dangerous to us than the illness it treats. It could also be termed *tough love health care*, which represents a willingness to address unpopular issues about the health care process and our role in it in order to improve outcome. This is a consumer advocate viewpoint.

A consumer point of view is decidedly different from a provider point of view. When health providers become health consumers, they are treated with the professional courtesy and deference usually extended to colleagues. Consumers receive no preferential treatment in the health care system, particularly in an environment of managed care. The opinions of providers are important, but theirs are not the only ones that matter. The opinions of consumers who have experienced health services firsthand are equally important and represent voices too rarely heard in health care.

Simplifying the Complex

The choices of alternative practices have become seemingly endless, and the information on them a virtual assault on the senses. There are thousands of books and more than two thousand magazines, journals and newsletters on alternative healing and related subjects, making it a publishing bonanza. Even people who have been using alternative medicine for a long time are daunted by its explosion in the media marketplace along with its intense promotion. What is daunting to the experienced user will certainly be intimidating to the novice.

There is so much information about alternative medicine that it is difficult to know what is reliable and what is not. Many publications are lengthy and laborious, spending fifty pages on what could be said in two and offering more detail and minutia than most people want or could possibly assimilate. Guides that claim to simplify alternative medicine make it even more complex by identifying and defining every alternative medicine system, modality, practice, therapy, or remedy ever created and offering encyclopedic lists of do's and occasional don'ts for its use.

You could easily spend thousands of dollars and several years before becoming competent enough to make informed choices about alternative medicine, a difficult task for a healthy person. When confronted with serious illness, spending a great deal of time, energy, and money exploring alternative medicine options is not very practical. Serious illness limits one's physical and emotional capacity for investigation, and high medical premiums and copayments preclude extensive additional expenditures. Wading through the complexities of alternative medicine at any time is a difficult task.

This guide is user-friendly, cutting through New Age rhetoric to reach the bottom line. Summaries of the main points and practical suggestions are offered throughout the guide. This *Cliff Notes™* approach simplifies alternative medicine without sacrificing an understanding of its complexity and the importance of using it safely and responsibly. It condenses the best alternative medicine has to offer into the most usable components. What is easier to understand is also easier to use. Instead of buying ten books on alternative medicine, you can get started on the right path with just one.

The Framework

Another example of making the complex clear is featured in the six-step plan which presents a framework or formula for using alternative medicine. It makes alternative medicine more accessible, organizing it in a simple and logical manner. The plan divides alternative medicine into steps that encompass lifestyle change, the balance of external and internal energy, our thought processes, physical restriction and limitation, and the protection of our bodies, minds, and souls.

Within each step are examples of alternative practices that reflect the identified goal. Once you choose a practice that best suits your needs, it is your responsibility to educate yourself about the practice. To assist you in this effort, suggested readings about the featured practices are offered throughout the six-step plan.

A Multi-Faceted Approach

A multifaceted approach to illness means using more than one practice at one time to achieve the best results. It is surprising that few alternative medicine proponents with their avowed holistic viewpoints encourage a multifaceted approach to health. There may be several reasons for this. Science studies the effectiveness of one technique or treatment modality at a time. Publications advocate one alternative practice or therapy because they are typically written by people who are trained in the practice or therapy. Not only do most alternative providers know little about practices other than their own, but they can also be proprietary about clients.

It does not make sense to put all your eggs in one basket, believing that one therapy or technique will facilitate a complete and permanent cure. A combination of therapies or techniques is usually necessary in order to bring the body back into a state of balance and harmony.

A Comprehensive Approach

A comprehensive approach to illness means considering all aspects of health at one time—physical, mental, and spiritual. There is much talk about the mental and spiritual in alternative medicine, but these aspects of health are frequently omitted from the actual treatment process. They are addressed in the six-step plan and include controversial practices such as *feng shui* and past life therapy.

There are also separate chapters about using psychotherapy, facilitating medical surgery, and changing attitudes about death and dying. We all know about the importance of maintaining healthy lifestyle habits, but no comprehensive approach to alternative medicine would be complete without their consideration as a precursor to its use.

The Bigger Picture

You cannot use alternative medicine with any degree of success unless you understand the bigger picture, the environment most conducive to true healing. Alternative medicine embraces a broader view of health and how illness is regarded and treated. In this view, health is a state of mind, so illness does not always include physical incapacitation or impairment. It is also a normal part of life from which the body, like nature, has a natural inclination to heal itself on its own without any intervention. In many cases, this is exactly what will happen.

Other times, the natural ability to heal may be inhibited because the body is overwhelmed by a variety of circumstances. When this occurs, alternative interventions, based on the belief that everything you need for healing is found in nature, are employed to encourage this natural ability. The alternative interventions that you choose depend on the underlying causes of your imbalance, and more than one is usually necessary to bring the body back into a state of balance. In alternative medicine, there are many facets to healing other than the use of medical intervention.

When an imbalance occurs, healing is more complex and takes more time to resolve than we think it should. It usually involves more than taking a pill, using a single remedy or technique, undergoing surgery to excise the problem, or finding an answer through scientific research. Healing that lasts necessitates assessment and intervention on many different levels and at different stages of the healing process. It also requires the active and full participation of the person who wishes to be healed. In order for alternative medicine to really be effective, we must change the way we view illness. In order to change the way we view illness, we must change the way we view the world.

Our definition of health and the purpose of medicine is much broader than what we were taught. It extends way beyond the limitations of our fears and egos and the definitions provided by medical science because there are aspects of health in a holistic perspective that science will likely never be able to validate. When we expand our awareness in this manner, we understand that our bodies are not the enemy and illness is a consequence, not a cause, of what ails us. Illness is merely wisdom struggling to attract our undivided attention.

Alternative medicine is based on the premise that you play an active role in the healing process. It encourages you to look deeper into the underlying basis for your illness instead of focusing on the immediate alleviation of symptoms. In doing so, you develop self-awareness and can circumvent potential health problems before they become more serious. The bottom line is that an involved, informed consumer raises the standards of any industry and is more likely to experience a positive outcome from the use of its goods or services. In alternative medicine, this outcome is healing.

Alternative medicine, like any external intervention, provides tools from the outside in order to facilitate healing on the inside. The use of alternative medicine does not guarantee health or the avoidance of illness. There is no such thing as a miracle drug or miracle treatment. There are only miracle people.

Health Care Crossroads

In the new millennium, our society is faced with serious global conflicts. Health care resources are unavailable to many people for a variety of reasons, and diverse, flexible, and culturally appropriate health strategies are sorely lacking. At the same time, the potential for healing ourselves through personal growth and creative change has never been greater. This potential is enhanced with the realization that the human being is more than a living machine, like an automobile, to be repaired by doctors who are trained to be more body mechanics than healers. In our complex world, a guide that promotes this view is simply an aid to survival.

CHAPTER 1

ALTERNATIVE VERSUS CONVENTIONAL MEDICINE

After decades of relative obscurity and clandestine use, alternative medicine has come out of the closet and is experiencing explosive growth in our society. We are only just beginning to touch the surface of our ability to improve our own health. As conventional medicine suffers from what appears to be an irreversible and potentially catastrophic economic crisis and a consumer revolt against its failure to adequately address our needs, alternative medicine has become socially acceptable in mainstream culture.

Education, science, and industry are all scrambling to jump on the bandwagon, and curiosity has replaced cynicism about the role alternative medicine plays in health care. Public opinion about alternative medicine has also dramatically changed. In some circles, the use of alternative medicine is considered chic, and constant references about what it can do for you are made in the national media.

Consumers want in on it because they are dissatisfied with the negative turns conventional medicine has taken in recent years and are looking for a better way to address their health concerns. Baby boomers want in on it because they believe that alternative medicine will delay or transform the aging process. Health providers want in on it because they are afraid of losing customers and their dollars. Insurance companies want in on it because the preventive focus of alternative medicine may reduce benefit payments.

The alternative medicine business—and it has clearly become one—generates billions of dollars every year in consumer spending for publications, products, and practitioners and covers everything from consciousness to healing to mysticism. The opportunity for both misperception and exploitation is ripe in such a growth-oriented industry. Concepts like holistic medicine and spirituality are trivialized by mass consumerism, creating a complex environment, which people must navigate at their own risk. Buddhist monks are used to sell automobiles, yoga is used to sell vodka, and meditators are used to sell everything from stock buying services to hamburgers. Alternative products are even sold via pyramid marketing programs like Amway.

The popularity of alternative medicine and the intense scrutiny it generates creates the potential for harm. Most people would agree that our health care system is in dire straits, and alternative medicine is now being added to this mix. *As it becomes slowly incorporated into our health care system, alternative medicine stands a good chance of acquiring many of the same problems that currently plague conventional medicine.* Institutionalized medicine is unresponsive to the needs of consumers, and commercialized medicine prioritizes profit over all other concerns. The integrity of alternative medicine is clearly threatened in this environment, creating a climate for possible misuse and abuse.

Surveys conducted in the past several years suggest that 50–70% of the population uses some form of alternative medicine every year, particularly for self treatment and chronic conditions. One study concludes that this constitutes more than 600 million visits to alternative practitioners, more than the number of visits to conventional doctors. Consumers spend an estimated $40 billion annually on alternative medicine. Disciplines like yoga are booming with an estimated 15 million participants, more than twice as many who were practicing five years ago. Another survey confirmed broad use of alternative medicine across age and demographic groups and its steady increase for the past fifty years.

There are many reasons why people use alternative medicine. Although there are those who use it because of their dissatisfaction with conventional treatment, others use alternative medicine because they believe that it will work and is consistent with their values, beliefs, and philosophical orientation toward health and life. Some people use it because they are health-conscious while others use it only after experiencing a serious health crisis.

Whatever the reason, there is an undeniable tolerance for alternative medicine that has never existed before. Conventional medicine is often described as "too much technology and not enough talk." Perhaps it is in this void that alternative medicine is gaining such widespread consumer support.

Definitions

Alternative medicine covers a wide range of healing therapies, methodologies, and philosophies. The National Center for Complementary and Alternative Medicine at the National Institutes of Health (NIH) defines alternative medicine as those health care practices *not* considered an integral part of conventional medicine. It has also been described as practices that are *not* widely taught in medical schools, generally used in hospitals, or usually reimbursed by medical insurance companies.

Alternative medicine is known as mind/body, holistic, complementary, integrated, Eastern, unconventional, traditional, or nontraditional medicine. Conventional medicine is often termed Western, standard, traditional, or allopathic medicine. Although some people are strident in their preference of one term over another, it is more important how you use it than what you call it. In this guide, health provider or practitioner refers to any provider of health services, including medical doctors.

Basic Differences

Conventional and alternative medicine represent opposite viewpoints, but they both have their place in health care. Instead of believing one is better than another, it is important to understand that they simply differ in their approach to health. These differences are delineated as follows:

Conventional Medicine	Alternative Medicine
1. science and technology	1. nature
2. business	2. art
3. disease and failure	3. prevention and success
4. absence of disease	4. healing
5. repair of structural systems in the body	5. enhancing the body's natural ability to heal itself
6. visible	6. visible and invisible
7. addresses one part of the at a body time	7. addresses the whole person

8. treats symptomatically

9. physical cause of disease

10. doctor opinion and beliefs

8. treats underlying causes of illness

9. physical, emotional, and spiritual cause of disease

10. consumer opinion and beliefs

Healers Versus Doctors

In ancient healing traditions, healers were a small and highly select group chosen at birth or an early age to develop what-was-perceived-as an innate healing ability. They were valued for their sensitivity and clarity of mind, technical skill, and purity of intention. Although held in high regard in their respective communities, healers were never wealthy. They usually possessed psychic gifts and the ability to address the invisible along with the visible. They made no distinction among physical, mental, and spiritual aspects of health and were doctors, psychologists, and priests all rolled into one. In these traditions, healing was considered to be an art.

Healers were usually compensated by barter or donation based on a person's ability to pay and his appreciation for the skill of the healer. In the Chinese medicine tradition, doctors were only paid as long as the client remained well. No fees were paid once a client became ill because the doctor was considered to have failed in his efforts. Although this approach gives more credit to the healer than it should, it does illustrate an emphasis on prevention rather than intervention. *This emphasis is completely reversed in our system of health care.*

Today, medicine is a business, and doctors are chosen on the basis of competitive academic scores, the ability to afford medical school, and the stamina to survive medical training. Medical schools choose candidates for their knowledge and potential skill, but clarity of mind and purity of intention are not standard selection criteria. Since training does not begin until adulthood, doctors spend more time working on others than on themselves. They are trained to be techno-interventionists, addressing only the visible and treating illness symptomatically in sterile office environments. In the conventional paradigm, doctors only profit when people are ill because this is the only time they seek medical attention. Since medical costs are so high, most doctors are quite wealthy.

Medical doctors are not typically trained to see a bigger picture beyond physical illness (or mental illness if they are psychiatrists). This limitation translates into "the blind leading the blind" from the holistic perspective. Although performing a successful surgery does not require a grasp of the meaning of life, helping a patient recover from it and heal properly does. The unconsciousness of modern medicine does little to promote or encourage healing over technical cure.

If modern medicine were an art, there would be far fewer doctors practicing today, and if the incomes of conventional doctors were dependent on keeping patients well, their livelihoods would be in serious jeopardy. Since medicine is a business and not an art, you must exercise the same caution toward alternative medicine that you would use to purchase any other product or service.

Negativity of Conventional Medicine

There are probably few of us who have not been subject to the negativity of conventional medical care. During my own health scare several years ago, I was given little chance of a complete recovery, refused an x-ray protective shield by a technician who told me that wearing one "didn't matter," denied vital information on an alternative remedy proven effective in a study conducted by one of my own doctors, and told that the negative effects of treatment on my reproductive system were unimportant because, at the age of 38, I was "too old to have a child."

As if that were not enough to contend with, I began receiving collection notices from an out-of-state attorney for bogus hospital visits with my primary care physician. A well-known university medical clinic made harassing phone calls to my home to collect monies for which I was not responsible. My insurance company tripled my rates, refusing to pay for treatment such as physical therapy, which they categorized in their denial as "personal fitness training," and threatening to cancel my policy if I did not return to work when I was completely immobilized.

I remember thinking that if the disease does not kill me, the medical system treating me surely will. Having to muster up the energy to respond to these negative incidents caused a diminishment of the resources I desperately needed to get well. An unsupportive atmosphere such as this is not conducive to healing and poses a far greater threat to your health than illness.

It is this medical environment to which we are subjected—some of us repeatedly—today. Is this what the Greek physician Hippocrates, widely believed to be the father of modern medicine, intended when he wrote, "As to diseases, make a habit of two things—to help, or at least to do no harm"?

Conventional doctors have inadvertently impeded the healing process with their negativity for a long time. Conventional medicine focuses on the treatment of disease over the facilitation of healing, restricting itself to the physical causes of illness. Doctors are notorious for being pessimistic prognosticators because they typically treat the worst cases of illness while fully recovered clients often do not return for examinations or follow-up care. Medical training encourages them to maintain a detached attitude, the antithesis of what clients need and want. Diagnoses are held in such high regard that people usually become their diseases. When a person recovers despite a doctor's negative predictions, either the diagnostic tests are declared inaccurate or the recovery is labeled an inexplicable "spontaneous remission." People are rarely given credit for their own ability to heal.

Women are frequent consumers of health services. Most women have probably been told at least once by a medical doctor that the problem for which they sought treatment is emotional or "in their heads" in a manner that is either dismissive or belittling. There are, however, emotional and spiritual aspects to every physical imbalance, so this narrow medical view not only demonstrates ignorance on the part of the doctor but disrespect for the totality of the individual. Any doctor who tells you to fix your attitude in such a manner frankly needs to fix his.

Conventional medicine's goal is the elimination of disease to ease suffering; however, this medicine and the system that supports it often increase suffering. They do this through preventable medical mistakes, the adverse and sometimes dangerous effects of prescription drugs, and the negative attitudes described above, which also create unnecessary stress. In many ways, modern medicine, with its techno-pharmacological focus, attempts to usurp the power we naturally possess to heal ourselves, even telling us when to live or die. Alternative medicine allows us to reclaim our power in this process.

Confusion of Alternative Medicine

Although conventional medicine has become incredibly negative, alternative medicine is equally confusing. There are an overwhelming number of alternative practices in the marketplace and enormous disagreement about what is reliable and effective. Within the practices themselves, there are conflicting viewpoints and insularity. There are new alternative practices that are slick on the surface but slack on substance. Many practices that claim to be holistic do not encourage wholeness in any form. The dizzying array of information on alternative medicine is exhaustive and exacerbates rather than alleviates the confusion.

Deciding on an alternative practice is only a first step. Once a practice is chosen, you must find a competent practitioner with whom a positive relationship can be built. Among alternative practitioners, there are huge variances in knowledge, skill level, training, experience, and expectations. Some guides to alternative medicine demand changes in lifestyle so extreme that you feel discouraged and inadequate if you are unable to make them. Ironically, this is the type of stressful atmosphere any responsible alternative provider will tell you is *not* conducive to healing.

There are thousands of alternative medicine remedies from which to choose in the herbal marketplace. More than one remedy addresses the same complaint, and a remedy or dosage that works for one person may not work in the same way for another person. Mail order companies, broadcast infomercials, and Internet websites feverishly market and promote the sale of natural remedies and supplements, which may or may not live up to claims. As a result of all this, many people choose to do nothing rather than deplete their already diminishing resources or make a serious mistake with their health.

Conventional Medicine in an Emergency

Conventional medicine is most effective addressing life-threatening or crisis medical conditions. Without medical technology, there would be no organ transplant, prosthetics, or reconstructive surgery. In crisis conditions, conventional medicine has an undeniable track record for saving lives.

The drugs used to treat crisis conditions are highly suppressive and toxic because they were designed to quickly attack and eradicate the acute, killer diseases of the nineteenth century. Unfortunately, these drugs are still being used to treat the chronic, aging illnesses of today, giving rise to the saying "If the disease doesn't kill you, the treatment will." The price paid for conventional treatment of illness is often incapacitating symptoms and the suppression and resulting breakdown of the body's natural immunity.

Conventional medicine sometimes involves the sacrifice of one organ to save another. Although justified in a life-threatening situation, this is a high price to pay for what are frequently only short-term results. In other instances, conventional medicine can increase the probability of incurring another disease. For example, synthetic estrogen supplementation increases the risk for breast and ovarian cancer as does chemotherapy for new cancerous growths. The statistics speak for themselves. Prescription drugs cause more than 100,000 deaths every year.

There are currently no alternatives to the invasiveness of conventional crisis care; however, alternative medicine can reduce many of its negative side effects. It can be used as an adjunct to conventional treatment to the extent that your time and pocketbook allow and with consideration for the effect of one medicine on the other. Conventional wisdom states that, for a major imbalance, the combined use of conventional and alternative medicine is probably warranted, but minor imbalances can usually be resolved with alternative medicine alone.

Alternative Medicine in a Non-Emergency

While conventional medicine is best in a crisis or life-threatening situation, alternative medicine is best in almost all other medical situations, which comprise the majority of illness. In noncrisis conditions, alternative treatment is not only more effective but less harmful to the body. If used properly, it takes into account every aspect of a person's life. Alternative medicine used preventively does not guarantee freedom from illness. It goes a long way, however, to preventing it and can greatly facilitate recovery if illness occurs.

Conventional drugs may work fast to suppress symptoms of illness, but their effect is often temporary, causing new symptoms of the same underlying problem to appear elsewhere in the body. Due to their natural sources, diluted natures, and ability to work with the body rather than against it, alternative remedies alleviate symptoms of illness safely and often permanently. For the most part, they are nonaddictive and produce negligible side effects if used properly. They also work much slower than conventional drugs, so a longer period of time is required in order to achieve results. Time is a small price to pay for physical safety and possible permanent resolution.

There is no question that it is easy to choose alternative medicine when you are faced with a minor injury or illness but more difficult to choose it when your life is at stake. There is more to lose if you do not get it right, and finding out what works and what does not work usually involves time-consuming trial and error.

When faced with a serious health crisis, there will probably be little support from your conventional doctor for using alternative medicine. The fact that these two systems of medicine are so polarized from one another creates an interesting dilemma. Conventional doctors frequently apply crisis medicine to noncrisis conditions, and alternative practitioners apply noncrisis medicine to undiagnosed crisis conditions.

Today, prescription drugs and surgery are the main focus of standard medicine with alternative methods employed only as a last resort. Someday, alternative methods and an emphasis on self-care will be the main focus of standard medicine with conventional drugs and surgery employed only as a last resort. This is the way it should be.

Insurance Benefits

Alternative medicine is more costly to use than conventional medicine because insurance companies do not pay benefits for it unless it is prescribed by medical doctors. One notable exception to this rule exists in the state of Washington, which passed a bill requiring insurance companies to pay for licensed or certified alternative medicine practitioners. Other states have followed with similar bills. Some medical doctors practice alternative medicine as their primary focus. Most insurance policies routinely pay for the services of osteopaths and chiropractors, but coverage for practices such as Chinese medicine, naturopathic medicine, and massage is less common or limited and varies from state to state and plan to plan.

This has both a good and bad side to it. A lack of insurance coverage for alternative medicine means that regulators have little control over what you choose, but it also means that you must pay for alternative medicine out of your own pocket. The latter may become prohibitive as costs for using alternative medicine rise with its increasing popularity.

Although attitudes are quickly changing, many insurance companies still believe that providing benefits for alternative medicine is more costly than supporting tried and true conventional methods. This is flawed thinking. Although more expensive in the short run, the preventive and nontechnological nature of alternative medicine will save money in the long run.

A New Vision

Current discussions about alternative and conventional medicine dwell on their differences, but there should be greater interest in how they can work together rather than work

Integrated Health Care System

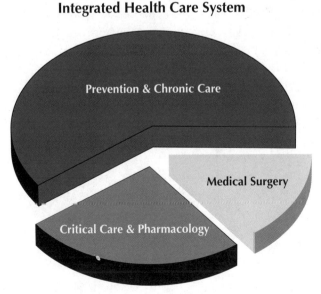

Fig. 1. Future Health Care System

against one another. It is easy to envision a future health care system in which there are three highly interactive branches: prevention and chronic care, critical care and pharmacology, and medical surgery (see Fig. 1).

The prevention and chronic care branch utilizes alternative medicine systems, methods, techniques, remedies, and psychological specialists and includes education and self-care. The critical care and pharmacology branch consists of the use of conventional and emergency medicine to address life-threatening illnesses, accidents, and other crisis conditions. The surgery branch involves emergency surgery, organ transplantation, and reconstruction with elective surgery regarded as a final option. Both the critical care and surgery branches work closely together with the prevention branch to enhance the recovery process and ameliorate the effects of conventional medicine techniques and drugs.

The emphasis in this system of medicine is clearly on prevention and maintaining a state of physical, mental, and spiritual balance before problems occur. Consumers are also given incentives to engage in regular prevention. Alternative medicine is applied to noncrisis conditions and used in conjunction with conventional medicine for crisis conditions. All health care services are available to consumers in one facility and in an environment that is warm, welcoming, and conducive to healing.

Choosing a Practitioner

Choosing an alternative practitioner is a complex process because of the variables involved and the fact that alternative practices are so different from one another in their orientation and approach, even within the same discipline. The differences can be significant. For example, some osteopaths practice primary care while others practice only hands-on bodywork. Some acupuncturists combine acupuncture with acupressure, others combine it with herbs, and others use acupuncture alone. There are numerous ways to practice massage. Read about the practice so you know what to expect.

If you live in an area where there are many alternative practitioners, consult with more than one, if possible, before making a decision. Talking with a practitioner on the phone or meeting him in an introductory consultation provides valuable information and can narrow your choices. Practical matters should also be considered such as making sure that the provider's fees, practice schedule, and office policy coincide with your needs. Some alternative providers will even make house calls if you are too ill to go to their office.

In order to make responsible choices about alternative providers, you must first get reliable referrals and then evaluate the qualifications and appropriateness of the practitioners who are recommended to you.

Referrals

Getting good referrals is the first step toward finding a good alternative practitioner. This is primarily a word-of-mouth business. Referrals for practitioners can come from a variety of sources. *The best source is from people you know and trust.* Other sources of referrals to alternative practitioners include:

- other consumers of alternative medicine
- conventional or alternative practitioners
- alternative medicine professional associations
- natural food stores and other natural health retail businesses
- alternative medicine schools and training programs
- support groups for medical conditions (i.e., diabetes, etc.)
- local New Age magazines and newspapers
- alternative medicine referral services (if available in your area)
- yellow pages of the telephone book
- public, university, and medical libraries
- advocacy group newsletters (i.e., Arthritis Foundation)
- outpatient hospital programs (i.e., stress management)
- the Internet
- health information research services
- health clubs (i.e., yoga classes or knowledgeable personal trainers)

Licenses

After getting a good referral, take the time to investigate the practitioner's credentials. Find out if the practitioner is licensed, and make sure his license is in good standing with the appropriate state licensing board. Licensing for alternative medicine practices varies from state to state but usually includes Chinese Medicine practitioners (OMD for doctor of oriental medicine or LAc for acupuncturist), homeopaths (DHM), naturopaths (ND), osteopaths (DO), and chiropractors (DC).

There are medical doctors (MD) who practice alternative medicine such as homeopathy, acupuncture, and nutritional medicine. Their training usually takes place as continuing or postgraduate education. Approximately 75 out of 117 medical schools in the United States now incorporate alternative medicine topics in required or elective courses.

There are many skilled alternative practitioners who are not licensed because the state does not issue or require a license or because they choose to be unlicensed. An alternative practitioner may also be unlicensed because the school from which he received his training does not meet the educational requirements of the state licensing board.

Certification in an alternative practice is not the same as a state license from a government-sanctioned board. Certifications are issued by the organizations that actually conduct the training, and these programs vary in quality from program to program and may only consist of a weekend workshop.

There are advantages and disadvantages to using a licensed alternative practitioner. When you use a licensed practitioner, you are assured some protection if the service you receive falls below the standard of care for the practice. On the other hand, licensing merely signifies that training and testing requirements of licensing boards are met and is not an absolute guarantee of competence.

Before an Appointment

There are several things you can do before scheduling an appointment with an alternative practitioner. Contact the provider to inquire about his approach to treatment, particular areas of expertise, where he trained, and how long he has been in practice. Find out if he has treated others with your condition and the results of their treatment. Ask him to send you a copy of his curriculum vitae (CV) or resume if he has one. A CV will indicate if he is a member of any professional associations. If so, contact them about his standing. Professional associations set standards for members and may revoke or suspend membership if standards are not met. Most professional associations maintain their own websites.

Alternative providers employ a variety of approaches to treatment. Some use a single modality while others combine different modalities together in the same practice. Examples of a singular approach are providers who practice orthomolecular medicine, which focuses on the use of vitamins and minerals; biological medicine, which focuses on the use of diet and other lifestyle issues; and herbal medicine, which focuses on the use of herbs. An example of an eclectic approach is a provider who practices orthomolecular and/or herbal medicine but, at the same time, uses detoxification therapies such as colonic irrigation, fasting or juicing, and chelation or vitamin C therapy. Most alternative providers have particular areas of expertise, and some specialize in treating certain health conditions.

Find out where the alternative provider received his training. There are a growing number of alternative medicine training programs cropping up all across the country. Some are little more than diploma mills, providing quick degrees or certifications to students for a fee and lasting only a few weeks. Others provide students with an authentic and comprehensive educational experience and require several years to complete. Contact the training program about their admission requirements and program of study to discover if it is the former or the latter. Most alternative medicine training programs also have websites.

The length of time a provider has practiced is also critical in the use of alternative medicine. It is usually, but not always, an indication of just how good a practitioner will be. Alternative practices are not learned quickly unless a person has a natural affinity for them. While such practitioners do exist, they are not on every street corner. Tibetan doctors are required to undergo intensive training, beginning in early childhood and lasting more than a decade, before being allowed to practice on their own. Most established alternative practices require years of training and experience before providers are considered proficient in the practice and see results in their work.

Face to Face Assessment

Once you confirm that a practitioner is properly trained and experienced, the only way to find out if you are compatible with him is through a face to face assessment. Sometimes, you can accomplish this in a brief introductory consultation, lasting anywhere from fifteen to twenty minutes, at no charge or a reduced fee.

Communication is the cornerstone of any good health care relationship, and practitioners should be willing and able to talk with you about any issue that affects your health,

no matter how unusual or intimate. They should be respectful, helpful, positive, supportive, easy to understand, and
good listeners, placing your interests first and encouraging
informed health care choices.

When you meet a practitioner face to face, you have a
better idea if he is the right one for you, but you can only
find out what he knows and how good he really is when you
receive treatment from him. This may take several sessions
because results take time with the use of alternative medicine. It also takes time to discover how truly committed a
practitioner is to your well-being.

Intentions are an important, but rarely considered, aspect
of treatment because motive affects outcome. A provider's primary motivation for practice can be honorable or superficial.
He may practice because he is committed to your health and
well-being or because he needs to feel important or in control.
Since the Western approach to medicine includes the belief
that the doctor is responsible for healing, it is important for an
alternative practitioner to realize that he is only a facilitator
and not the source of healing. He must be in harmony with
himself about his collaborative role in order to truly help you.

As with any health provider, alternative practitioners
have either good intentions or misplaced ones, and they possess skill levels that are excellent, mediocre, or poor. With
these criteria in mind, you can divide alternative practitioners into three basic groups:

1. Practitioners who are well intentioned and highly
   skilled who want positive, equitable relationships with
   patients. These practitioners are the most in demand
   and the most difficult to find.

2. Practitioners who are well intentioned with average
   or poor skill. A positive relationship with this

practitioner may compensate for a lack of ability, but it can also be a waste of time and money, especially if he does not know what he is doing.

3. Practitioners who practice for reasons other than to facilitate your healing and place their interests above that of your own, very often unconsciously. These practitioners may be highly skilled, but skill does not compensate for poor motives because you can be hurt as much by a practitioner's intent as you can his lack of skill.

Caveats

Many people become alternative practitioners solely because of their own personal experiences with illness and healing through the use of alternative medicine. Although it is helpful to have a practitioner with firsthand experience, *healing oneself is very different from healing others.* Just because a person can do one does not necessarily mean that he can do the other. Training and education provide practitioners with the necessary technical skill, but alternative practitioners who are popular and achieve consistently positive results seem to possess an innate capacity for healing that existed long before attending any training or educational program.

There are alternative practitioners whose work is holistic in theory but not in practice. Some practitioners use the increasingly popular catchphrase "body, mind, and spirit" loosely without knowing what it means in the context of your health or how to apply it in actual practice. They may do this to impress you with their knowledge of alternative concepts, but this does not always denote a genuine understanding of the phenomenon and how it works. For some reason, people feel better hearing it and alternative providers feel better saying it. Embracing the concept is not the same as being able to practically apply it to your care, and claiming that it is the basis of an alternative practice does not necessarily make it so.

There is a gross assumption that all alternative practitioners are above reproach because of the altruistic basis of alternative medicine. *This is a huge misconception.* In fact, the intangible nature of alternative medicine actually makes it *more* difficult to spot a fraud or an incompetent practitioner. People with serious health conditions often blind themselves to this reality because they are desperate for answers. But people are people in any profit-making profession. When the profession involves the potential loss of your health or life, however, the stakes are much higher.

Enormous competition exists among the many alternative practices for your consumer dollar. This competitive environment can discourage referrals to other providers. For this reason, you must exercise vigilance about your progress and know when it is time to discontinue a relationship with an alternative provider. Be wary of practitioners who keep you coming for regular visits without any noticeable sign of improvement or reasonable explanation about the status of your condition. This is a sure sign that you need to move on.

Be Proactive

The key to getting the most from an alternative practitioner is to assume a proactive approach by being assertive and fully involved in your care. This approach is the basis for my book, *Is Your Health Care Killing You? 12 Ways to Survive Our Fractured Health Care System*, and applies to both conventional and alternative medicine. Responsible alternative practitioners will encourage you to pursue this approach because the successful use of alternative medicine depends on it. A proactive approach not only improves your chances for healing but also makes their job easier.

Prepare for your visit by writing down the issues you want to discuss, and take it with you to your appointment. Be sure to identify your greatest concern at the beginning of the visit, not at the end. Ask lots of questions, and do not be satisfied with vague or incomplete answers. Be honest about any bad health habits. Insist on complete disclosure about alternative treatments and remedies and their risks or adverse reactions.

Find out what you can do to facilitate treatment, and do it. Be willing to monitor your progress by keeping track of changes in your condition. Assessment primarily depends on your experience with treatment rather than the results of diagnostic tests.

If diagnostic tests are employed, be sure to get copies of the results from your practitioner and ask him to explain them to you. Be willing to research health conditions and treatments on your own, and ask your practitioner for sources of reliable health information. Always check out information with your practitioner before using it. Find out if there other treatments or practices that would be more effective at addressing your needs. If you disagree with a treatment recommendation, say so and explain why you feel this way.

Problems with Practitioners

Problems can and do arise in relationships with alternative practitioners. They can be handled in one of three ways:

1. If you value the relationship, discuss the problem openly with the practitioner in order to seek a

mutually beneficial resolution. Try to do this in a way that does not put you or the practitioner on the defensive.

2. Terminate the relationship with the practitioner. You are under no obligation to continue seeing any alternative practitioner, especially if you are paying for treatment on your own. Treatment records are easily transferred to a new practitioner with a simple written request.

3. If the service provided falls below the standard of care for the alternative practice or injury results from negligence, incompetence, or misconduct, file a complaint against the practitioner with the appropriate licensing board and professional association. Complaints such as these should not be submitted to disciplinary agencies without careful consideration of the consequences to all parties. In the event of a serious problem, however, filing a complaint is as much a service to other consumers as it is in your own interests.

Other Considerations

There is no encompassing organization or association that includes every practitioner of alternative medicine (like the American Medical Association for conventional medical doctors) and no overall standard of care for alternative practices. The differing approaches in alternative medicine, even within the same practice, do not lend themselves to a single organizing association. Instead, there are numerous alliances in alternative medicine and associations of medical doctors who practice alternative medicine. (See Appendix A.)

Depending on where you live, there may be little support for your use of alternative medicine. Many conventional doctors still believe that alternative medicine does not work, and others think it will interfere with conventional treatment. Those who disparage its use usually do so because they have no experience with it, not because they know it will not help you.

Although studies have shown that the majority of people (more than 60%) do not disclose their use of alternative medicine to their medical doctors, you should keep your doctor informed about any activity that affects your treatment. Insist that your alternative and conventional providers work closely together to provide you with better, more comprehensive care. When you demand excellence in your health providers, you have a better chance of receiving it. Providers are better providers when people are better consumers.

Alternative medicine is a business like any other, so choosing an alternative practitioner requires the same preparation and scrutiny you would use to purchase any product or service. Although there are obvious caveats to keep in mind to avoid the disreputable ones, there are many qualified practitioners of alternative medicine. In fact, what makes any alternative practice unique are the innate skills and talents the practitioner brings to it. The manner in which you choose and use an alternative practitioner can discourage or maximize the success of your entire health care regimen.

SUMMARY & FURTHER READING

The Lost Art of Healing, Bernard Lown, M.D.

New Age Capitalism: Making Money East of Eden, Kimberly Lau

1. Get referrals to alternative practitioners from people you know or trust. Try to consult with more than one practitioner before making a decision.

2. If the practitioner has a license or professional membership, make sure it is current and in good standing.

3. Before scheduling an appointment, find out where the practitioner received training and how long he has practiced. Has he treated others with your condition, and if so, what was the outcome?

4. Determine whether you are compatible with the practitioner. Is he willing to assume a collaborative role and able to address all aspects of health—physical, mental, and spiritual?

5. Assess the practitioner's intentions for practice. Is his primary concern your welfare or is it something other than your welfare?

6. Assume a proactive approach to treatment—get involved and learn as much as possible about your condition and treatment.

7. Assess the practitioner's knowledge and skill. Is there improvement in your condition after giving the treatment or medicine enough time to work?

8. Be prepared to discontinue the relationship with a practitioner if it does not benefit you or serve your needs.

Alternative Medical Associations

American Holistic Medical Association
(505) 292–7788

American Holistic Health Association
(714) 779–6152

American Association for Health Freedom
(800) 230–2762

American Medical Women's Association
(703) 838–0500

American Holistic Nurses Association
(800) 278–2462

Society of Behavioral Medicine
(608) 827–7267

Complementary-Alternative Medical Association
(404) 284–7592

American Board of Holistic Medicine
(808) 572–4616

CHAPTER 3

How to Choose & Use
a Psychotherapist

When you are confronted with illness, not only the body but the mind can be overwhelmed by a variety of factors. The mind, like the body, has the natural ability to protect and heal itself on its own but may need support or an outside intervention in order to do so. As a result of this need, along with our desire for a more holistic approach to health, the use of psychotherapy is becoming increasingly popular in the treatment of physical disease. Psychotherapy is a building block of bodymind work because health begins with whom you are and what you think, say, and do. Psychotherapy can also help you deal with past wounds, which can be obstacles to growth, awareness, and ultimately healing.

Many experts believe that at least 80% of illness is psychosomatic. Researchers have found brain receptors responsible for thought and action throughout the body, suggesting that beliefs affect every cell in the body. The majority of people now accept the fact that the mind plays a major role in affecting overall health. Many techniques used to address this phenomenon are only available through the practice of psychotherapy. Psychotherapists have led the way in developing, utilizing, and promoting many of the bodymind techniques described in *Step Four* of the six-step plan.

Although we are now aware of the influence of mind and spirit on the body, these aspects of health are often disregarded or ignored in treatment. Conventional providers tend to be uncomfortable with these issues because they are not trained to deal with them. Although psychospiritual issues are an integral part of alternative medicine, many alternative practitioners also fail to address them in treatment, knowing more about them in theory than in practice. While doctors and other health practitioners have become caretakers of the body, psychotherapists have clearly become caretakers of the soul.

Why do we have separate professions for mind, body, and spirit if they are truly inseparable from one another? Ancient healers considered physical, psychological, and spiritual aspects of health at one time. At the very least, health practitioners would provide people with more complete care, maximizing the effectiveness of any medicine, if they would work collaboratively with psychotherapists. Not only would this result in better care, but it would also go a long way to eliminating the stigma that continues to be attached to psychotherapy.

Choosing a Psychotherapist

To choose a psychotherapist, you can easily adapt the same criteria listed in the previous chapter for choosing an alternative practitioner. Among health providers, therapists are the most likely to see you for a brief, introductory consultation at no charge or a reduced fee. Although compatibility is an important criterion for choosing any health provider, it is crucial in a relationship with a psychotherapist. The success of treatment is based entirely on how well you communicate with one another. If you cannot communicate with a therapist, you are simply wasting your time. Introductory consultations are an asset in this regard, allowing you to consult with more than one therapist at little or no cost before making a decision.

Psychotherapists vary considerably in their therapeutic approach to practice, their skill level, and the techniques they employ. This is another reason to consult with more than one therapist before making a decision. Every therapist has a different style that is unique to him. By consulting with more than one therapist, you gain insight into what to expect and what to avoid in therapy and you will ultimately be pointed in the direction of the therapist who can best serve your needs.

There are many psychotherapists, more in some locations than in others. Try to avoid finding one through the yellow pages. Again, personal referrals from people whom you know and trust and who are familiar with the therapist's skill and experience are essential in choosing wisely. Ask your health provider for his recommendations.

You also may need different therapists for different conditions, techniques, and levels of healing, so finding the right one can be a fluctuating commodity, requiring frequent assessment on your part. Keep in mind that this growth process may or may not be encouraged by the therapist with whom you initiate treatment. Finding the right therapist with the right skills and for the right circumstance is only slightly less difficult than finding the right mate.

Theoretical Approach & Techniques

Psychotherapy is a complex practice with many factors to consider before making a decision. Every psychotherapy practice is based on a primary theoretical viewpoint. Theoretical viewpoints for psychotherapy include psychoanalytical, psychodynamic, developmental, behavioral, cognitive, Gestalt, humanistic, existential, family systems, and transpersonal or psychospiritual. Some viewpoints are based on what is wrong with you while others are based on what is right. Find out the theoretical viewpoint of the therapist, what it means, and how it pertains to your particular situation or condition. Some therapists also specialize in treating people with certain health conditions such as traumatic stress or cancer.

Transpersonal psychotherapy is a relatively new theoretical viewpoint that considers experiences beyond the personal and includes issues such as consciousness and altered states of awareness. It addresses phenomena such as telepathy, precognition, visitations with angels or spirits, out-of-body experiences, and visions. Transpersonal therapists are trained to go beyond traditional talking therapy and view their clients in a more holistic manner. Hypnosis, guided imagery, breathwork, meditation, and journal writing are some of the many techniques that are utilized in transpersonal practice.

Some transpersonal therapists engage in somatic bodywork, a form of psychotherapy that seeks to resolve emotional patterns and conflicts through physical release in conjunction with or in place of verbal expression. There are also transpersonal psychotherapists who claim to be faith healers and spiritual mystics. Although it is certainly possible for a licensed therapist to possess paranormal or psychic skill, this claim can be more about a therapist's intentions and philosophical beliefs than his actual ability.

Altered states of awareness and other levels of consciousness are still widely regarded as mental illness or serious pathology by traditional therapists, but transpersonal therapists are trained to regard these experiences more tolerantly, as a normal part of everyday existence. In 1994, the American Psychiatric Association recognized spiritual problems as a condition for which people might seek therapy. As a result of this recognition, therapists may be more inclined to approach these issues with an open and balanced view.

There are hundreds of techniques used in psychotherapy: play therapy, dream analysis, role playing, hypnosis, guided imagery, meditation, breathwork, writing therapy, eye movement desensitization and reprocessing (EMDR), neuro-linguistic programming (NLP), biofeedback, regression therapy, and many others. Some techniques are considered to be conventional; others are regarded as alternative with a bodymind orientation. Some therapists specialize in only one technique, while others are trained to use a variety of techniques. There are also therapists who use no techniques whatsoever in practice other than traditional talking therapy.

Find out what techniques a therapist uses and their appropriateness for your situation. Ask the therapist if he has treated other clients with your condition and what the results were. Sometimes, it is helpful to read about a therapeutic technique, but other times knowing too much about one can diminish its effectiveness. Therapists can either provide you with information about techniques or explain why it is inappropriate for you to know more until the conclusion of therapy. Therapists can also recommend books on your condition and guides to bodymind medicine. Avoid therapists who resist your desire to know more about your condition and treatment.

Types of Psychotherapists

There are many types of psychotherapists. They include psychologists and psychiatrists who, by virtue of their training, are oriented toward the traditional medical model of diagnosis and treatment of disease. The traditional medical model is based on diagnosing a mental illness or condition and treating it with therapy and/or medication. For this reason, psychiatrists and psychologists tend to be more concerned with what is wrong with you than what is right. Counselors or counseling psychologists employ a more holistic approach to therapy based on a wellness model, which emphasizes mental health over mental illness.

Marriage and family therapists are oriented toward the dynamic of the family unit. Social workers emphasize the need to understand people in their social and cultural environments and the importance of using therapy, activism, policy change, and advocacy to help others. There are therapists with special areas of expertise such as child therapy or health psychology. Sports therapists help professional athletes improve performances. Industrial-organizational therapists work with staffing and workforce development of companies. Two fairly new types of therapists are market therapists, who help investors handle financial gains and losses from the stock market, and animal therapists.

Only psychiatrists, by virtue of their medical degree, can prescribe psychotropic medication such as antidepressants, although psychologists have lobbied for this privilege for years. Psychiatrists who restrict their practice to medication prescription and management are known as psychopharmacologists and provide little or no traditional therapy.

Frequently, medication is over-prescribed because psychiatrists acquiesce to client demands or feel compelled to alleviate their own discomfort with a client's condition.

Although psychotropic drugs are often misused as a bio-chemical replacement for facing painful emotional issues, there are also issues that cannot be adequately or properly addressed until a biochemical imbalance is corrected. With the exception of conditions involving significant impaired functioning, psychotropic drugs should only be used sparingly and temporarily.

Sometimes, therapists will ask you to take psychological tests that they administer themselves or through a testing specialist. If the therapist tests you himself, make sure he is qualified to both administer the test and interpret the results because training and experience is required to do this competently. Many tests are scored subjectively and can pose problems if the testing administrator or specialist has unresolved issues of his own. Psychological testing should only be conducted in the presence of a problem that cannot be assessed by direct observation in the interview process or severe impaired functioning.

Licenses & Fees

There are many licenses to practice psychotherapy, which vary from state to state. They include professional counselors (LPC), mental health counselors (MHC), marriage and family therapists (MFT or MFCC), clinical social workers (LCSW), clinical or counseling psychologists (PhD), and psychiatrists (MD). Some states allow the practice of psychotherapy without a license. In states where a license is required, unlicensed psychotherapists must identify themselves with alternate titles like grief counselor or hypnotherapist.

A therapist must be licensed in order for his clients to qualify for insurance benefits, although benefits are typically limited to a specific number of sessions per year. As with any health provider, a psychotherapy license only ensures the completion of training and testing requirements by state licensing boards and does not guarantee competence.

There are now hundreds of psychotherapy schools in this country. Although it is difficult to get a license to practice medicine, most anyone with a college degree and sufficient funds for training can get a license to practice psychotherapy.

Psychotherapy fees are based on three main criteria: (1) the experience and skill of the therapist, (2) the license held by the therapist, and (3) consumer demand for therapy services. Socially conscious therapists typically offer a sliding fee scale, based on your ability to pay, instead of charging a flat fee. Some therapists will allocate a percentage of therapy hours to low-paying clients and offer significant discounts on fees. Therapists tend to be the most negotiable of all health care practitioners because the competition is fierce, so take advantage of their flexibility.

If psychotherapists are caretakers of the soul and spirituality should not be for sale, charging fees for such services would be considered inappropriate in many cultures. Spiritual teachers from the East are compensated through voluntary giving called *dana*, or donations, which encourages the development of generosity and kindness on the part of the receiver. *Dana* can also include offerings other than money as long as there is genuine appreciation on the part of the giver. In this way, spiritual teachings are given value without being denied to anyone.

The mere suggestion of therapy by donation would no doubt cause heart palpitations in the ranks of therapists in the West, but this policy would go a long way toward separating the good from the bad therapists. Therapy by donation is also antithetical to the basis for conventional medicine, from which the practice of psychotherapy is derived.

In the late nineteenth century, the field of psychology was born out of the omission of mental health from conventional medical practice and the failure of an increasingly secularized religion to address psychospiritual problems. Like its predecessor, psychotherapy is a business and more about profit than healing art.

Professional Psychotherapy Schools

One of the main reasons it is so easy to acquire a license to practice psychotherapy is the growing number of professional psychotherapy schools. Professional psychotherapy schools are typically privately owned businesses for profit whose income is derived primarily from expensive tuition and fees. Typically, they are not eligible for publically funded research grants and receive little or no financial support from state governments.

The quality of education and training provided at professional schools varies enormously. Some schools are little more than correspondence schools and diploma mills, selling academic degrees for a fee. This is why it is so important to ask a therapist where he was trained. Those who resist divulging this information may have attended a less-than-reputable clinical program.

Not only does the quality of the education and training vary, but professional psychotherapy schools frequently lack the institutional and program accreditations of other schools, which can adversely affect a graduate's ability to secure a license to practice or get a job. On the other hand, professional schools sometimes provide students with a more progressive curriculum than traditional university programs, offering specializations in nontraditional areas of study such as health psychology or transpersonal psychology.

Although professional schools accept older students against whom university programs notoriously discriminate, they can be lax on admission requirements, failing to adequately screen candidates for eligibility. Students of all ages who are rejected by university programs are usually admitted to professional schools.

Professional therapy schools have created a glut of therapists in the marketplace. In some locations, there may even be more therapists than clients. Explosive growth in the psychotherapy field has had several outcomes, both positive and negative. Competition for clients lowers fees for service, making therapy more affordable and, consequently, available to more people. It also makes therapists less inclined to refer clients to other therapists and lowers ethical standards for practice.

A therapist who fails to return your calls outside the office is not likely to improve his priorities in the office. One therapist reportedly began a telephone conversation with an established client by curtly demanding, "What do you want!" If a therapist treats you in a rude or disrespectful manner, find another therapist. Not only is this behavior unprofessional, but it is also potentially harmful in a crisis situation. There are too many caring therapists for you to waste your time on those who are not.

Other Criteria

Many people find it difficult to ascertain competence in a psychotherapist because of the intangibility of therapy practice. For example, it is easier to know when a medical doctor administers the wrong drug than when a therapist administers the wrong message. Like any health provider, good therapists demonstrate a natural affinity and talent for their work long before attending psychotherapy school, which only serves to develop and enhance their innate ability.

A frequent and all-too-true joke in psychotherapy circles is that therapists choose the profession to fix themselves. Although self-exploration is certainly a healthy trait in any person and you want to find a therapist who has not lived life in a glass bubble, you should choose a therapist who has worked through his problems rather than one who seeks to work them out on you. No client should ever have to deal with the problems of the therapist. Therapy should never exist to serve the therapist's emotional or financial needs, although this unfortunate situation is all too common.

In 1993, the *American Psychologist* reported that almost 50% of individuals who seek help from a therapist do so for interpersonal relationship problems. Feeling displaced or estranged from family and friends is unfortunately a reoccurring theme in our society as work, job relocation, divorce, and technology hold such a prominent place in our lives. Many people seek out therapy to substitute for these important relationships and to replace the intimacy and friendship that are missing from their lives.

If this is your goal, you should choose a therapist who has the ability to see what is right as much as what is wrong with your life. Therapists trained in the wellness model are more likely to embrace this view than those trained in the traditional medical model of disease. Even so, therapists in general tend to pathologize clients because the science of psychology is based on the notion that human nature is inherently flawed or negative. Although many therapists use the traditional model, more and more of them recognize the positive side of human nature and the natural tendency for people to resolve their problems if given the appropriate tools and sufficient emotional support.

Recognizing the importance of seeing clients in their natural environment, some therapists will conduct sessions in your home instead of having you come to an office. There in a distinct advantage to this approach. Therapists can get to the relevant issues quickly and deduce the therapeutic techniques most likely to facilitate progress, saving you both time and money. This is an important, underutilized tool in psychotherapy, and more therapists should be willing to engage in this practice.

Your Therapeutic Rights

State licensing boards for psychotherapy set standards for practice for their licensees. Professional associations such as the American Psychological Association and American Counseling Association have ethical codes that members must follow. Licensing boards and professional associations can tell you whether a therapist is in good standing or if disciplinary actions have been taken against him. Information about standards is frequently available on the Internet or can be requested directly from the appropriate board and association.

Psychotherapy clients are entitled to certain rights, which are typically protected by state licensing boards and professional associations. The following therapeutic rights are taken from the brochure *Professional Therapy Never Includes Sex*, which states that you have the right to:

1. Receive information about the therapist's licensure, education, training, experience, professional association membership, specialization, and limitations.

2. Receive written information about fees, method of payment, insurance reimbursement, number

of sessions, substitutions (in cases of vacation or emergencies), and cancellation policies before beginning therapy.

3. Receive information about confidentiality and privilege and with whom your therapist will discuss your case.

4. Receive respectful treatment in a safe environment.

5. Ask questions about your therapy or refuse to answer any question or engage in any treatment.

6. Receive information about your progress including a summary of your therapy file, which you can transfer to any therapist you choose. Many states allow you to receive a copy of your mental health records, although the therapist may be allowed to withhold them from you if he believes that seeing them will cause you harm.

7. Get a second opinion about your therapy or the therapist's methods.

8. Report unethical or illegal behavior by a therapist.

9. End treatment without obligation or harassment.

Ending Treatment

If you do not notice some improvement within a few months of beginning psychotherapy, it is appropriate to question the direction of it. Do not hesitate to request a referral to another therapist if your therapist is clearly not helping you. Therapy is supposed to encourage growth and change, not prevent you from moving forward. Good therapists will recognize when therapy has stalled and not allow it to happen. They will also refer you to another therapist without your having to ask. If you do not have a good therapist, you will need to recognize this for yourself.

There is also a saying in psychotherapy that "analysis is paralysis." This means that you can become too dependent on therapy and analyze your problems to the extent that you are prevented from making decisions, taking responsibility, or owning the experiences in your life. Therapy can become an emotional rut into which you tumble without notice, and extracting yourself from it can be even more difficult than the original problem for which you sought help in the first place. Socrates said, "The unexamined life is not worth living." On the other hand, the overexamined life may not allow you to live.

Fifty years ago, people did not openly talk about their problems because it was considered in bad taste to do so. Today, the pendulum has definitely swung the other way, but so much so that we have created a national addiction to analyzing our problems to the sacrifice of other aspects of our lives. Witness the dearth of media pundits who dissect and speculate on just about everything from politics to movies to health. This addiction has created a culture of narcissism in the service of our egos, but *the goal of therapy is to engage in self-reflection without it becoming self-obsession.*

Sometimes, it is difficult to end a relationship with a therapist, particularly one who needs the business. Some therapists will aggressively pursue you to get you to stay in treatment. This is appropriate if ending treatment will cause you serious harm. In the absence of such a risk, however, this pursuit is a sign that the therapist needs you more than you need him.

As with any health provider, legitimate, serious complaints about the professional misconduct of a psychotherapist should be directed to the appropriate licensing board and professional association(s).

Is Therapy Right for You?

Psychotherapy is not a panacea for all your emotional troubles. It is only one of many tools to facilitate growth and transformation and, as such, is not right for everyone. On the surface, it is a little odd to pay a lot of money to tell your feelings to a stranger who knows you in no other context of your life and who may not have figured out any of his own problems. But therapy has become a necessary commodity in a culture of individualism, even though it is a poor substitute for close personal relationships.

A famous but controversial study conducted in 1952 by renowned psychologist Hans Eysenck found that therapy in general helped no more than the passage of time. My own clinical psychology mentor made the following claim about therapy: 30% results in improvement, 30% makes the problem worse, and 30% results in no change whatsoever, while the remaining 10% floats somewhere among the three categories.

Psychotherapy is overrated in our society because it has become so easy to get a license to practice and very few people are really good at it. For the most part, therapy practice is based on converting the innate talents of visionaries such as Carl Jung and Milton Erickson into techniques that others can emulate. You may be able to imitate the style of a person, but you can never actually be that person. Trying to translate a person's innate ability into a technique others can mimic will always cause an ingredient in the process to be missing.

A cultural addiction to analysis and an attachment to our emotional wounds are the primary reasons traditional talking therapy remains so popular. There are, however, many ways to "skin the same cat" that are less expensive and less fraught with peril. In fact, the most profound tools for growth and transformation involve silence rather than talk. You can achieve equal or greater results with techniques such as meditation, guided imagery, breathwork, and somatic bodywork. For this reason, psychotherapy is only a useful first step in the personal growth process. It can involve more if you are able to find a therapist who is trained to go beyond traditional talking therapy, helping you develop insight and awareness in more expansive ways.

You cannot substitute therapy for either intimacy or friendship, although it is frequently used for this purpose. Therapy constitutes a professional, not a personal, relationship. Insights can be gained from it, however, which you can then use to establish more meaningful relationships outside the therapeutic environment. If you lose yourself in the identity of a therapist or if the therapist has an unresolved personal agenda, you will lose your way instead of finding it. Psychotherapists do not have the answers to your problems; they merely have tools to help you find your own answers. No matter what anyone tells you, you must ultimately do the work yourself.

Psychotherapy can be a valuable and positive intervention for those who use it wisely. Remember that, as with any professional health care relationship, it is possible to defer to the expertise of a therapist without giving up control of your therapy. Responsible therapists encourage an equal partnership in the therapeutic process and will work collaboratively with other health providers in a cooperative effort to assist you in your healing journey.

SUMMARY

1. Get referrals to psychotherapists from people you know or trust. Try to consult with more than one therapist before making a decision.

2. If the therapist has a license or professional membership, make sure it is current and in good standing.

3. Before scheduling an appointment, find out where the therapist was trained, his theoretical viewpoint, his areas of expertise, and the therapeutic techniques he uses in treatment. Has he treated others with your condition, and if so, what was the outcome?

4. Determine whether you are compatible with the therapist. Are you comfortable talking to him about your problems?

5. Assess the therapist's motivation for practice. Does he practice psychotherapy to help you or to fix himself?

6. Assume a proactive approach to therapy—get involved and familiarize yourself with the bodymind concept.

7. Determine the therapist's knowledge and skill. Is there positive change in your condition within a few months of initiating therapy?

8. Be prepared to discontinue the relationship with the therapist if it does not benefit you or serve your needs.

Psychotherapy Associations

American Psychiatric Association
(703) 907–7300

American Psychological Association
(202) 336–5500

American Counseling Association
(703) 823–9800

National Association of Social Workers
(202) 408–8600

American Association for Marriage and Family Therapy
(202) 452–0109

Association for Humanistic Psychology
(510) 769–6495

Association for Transpersonal Psychology
(650) 424–8764

Society for Spirituality and Social Work
(607) 777–4603

United States Association for Body Psychotherapy
(202) 446–1619

International Somatic Movement Education and Therapy
Association (212) 229–7666

CHAPTER 4

HOW TO CHOOSE & USE AN ALTERNATIVE MEDICINE REMEDY

There are so many alternative medicine remedies in the marketplace that it is almost impossible for the uneducated consumer to know what to choose or how to use them safely, responsibly, and effectively. Most remedies are made from plants that possess medicinal properties; however, you do not need a prescription to get one or a doctor's advice to use one. It is easy for anyone to buy and use alternative remedies, but it is unwise to do so without taking the time to learn some basic facts. This is serious medicine, even though it is natural medicine, because there is still the potential for harm and misuse.

Alternative medicine remedies come in a variety of products and forms. They include nutritional supplements, Western herbs, Eastern herbs (i.e., Chinese herbs), essential oils, flower essences, and homeopathic remedies among others. They come in creams, oils, gels, powders, granules, liquids, extracts, tinctures, tonics, tablets, capsules, gelcaps, syrups, liniments, salves, patches, sprays, soups, teas, and herbs in their natural state. Herbal formulas can be made from the leaf, root, flower, seeds, bark, stems, and fruit. Herbs have primary functions, which are described as an anti-inflammatory, stimulant, diuretic, astringent, analgesic, sedative, antiseptic, etc.

Alternative remedies are no longer just found in natural food stores. Everyone has access to them. They are sold in grocery stores, pharmacies, plant nurseries, on radio and TV, by mail order, on the Internet, and almost anywhere else you can imagine. The quality of the remedy is more important than where you buy it, as is its proper application. Alternative remedies are now so popular that they are generically prescribed for every health condition imaginable.

One of the biggest problems with alternative remedies is that people want to use them on their own without educating themselves about the herbs or consulting with a qualified herbalist or botanical specialist. There may be several reasons for this: the lack of time for proper investigation and evaluation; a wish to avoid the cost of consultations, which are typically not covered by insurance policies; the need for more personal control over health care; and frustration with providers who are unable or unwilling to address their client's needs. Using alternative remedies without proper preparation and education, however, may result in harm and misuse and impact the overall effectiveness of the remedy.

A Complex Process

There are many variables and considerations in choosing the right alternative remedy, especially for medicinal purposes. You must first find the right remedy to address your particular condition. This entails assessment on a physical, emotional, and spiritual level. You then choose the form and strength of the remedy or herb that best suits your needs. Once these decisions are made, you must choose among dozens of different brands of the same remedy in a variety of formulas and combinations with the knowledge that alternative remedies vary enormously in quality and potency, depending on the manufacturer and manufacturing process.

How herbs are harvested, extracted from the plant, processed, stored, and packaged varies from manufacturer to manufacturer, affecting freshness and potency. Some remedies are standardized, and some are not. Alternative remedies can be made from only one part of the plant, the whole plant, or different parts of the same plant combined together. Some remedies contain only one herb; others contain a variety of herbs and ingredients in differing strengths.

After you have chosen the remedy, you must determine the appropriate dosage and length of treatment. Once you begin taking it, you must know when the remedy is having an adverse effect on you, so you can discontinue treatment.

It does not stop here. Typically, there is more than one remedy or herb that addresses the same health complaint. Although the use of a singular herb or remedy may easily resolve a health condition, different remedies are often required at different levels or stages of healing. Some remedies may be season-specific, most effective during certain times of the year. One of the trickiest parts about using alternative remedies is that the same dosage of the same remedy for the same condition may actually work differently for each person who uses it.

Despite their gentle natures, alternative remedies are easily misused. There are alternative remedies that are toxic in high doses. Some remedies should not be used in the presence of certain health conditions such as pregnancy; others must be taken on an empty stomach or at specific intervals in order to work properly. Alternative remedies can adversely interact with conventional drugs or other herbal remedies.

Unhealthy lifestyle habits such as poor nutrition or unman-
aged stress alter the effectiveness of alternative remedies.
While misuse may not always result in actual harm, it can
negate the effectiveness of the remedy.

Figuring all this out is difficult to do on one's own. A
great deal of time and expense is required for what is often
a trial and error process. A qualified herbalist or botanical
specialist can greatly expedite this process. An experienced
herbalist helps you zero in on the right remedy in a shorter
period of time and can detect obstacles to using a remedy
or herb before it causes a more serious problem. In many
instances, the cost of finding the right remedy on your own
far outweighs the cost of one or two herbal consultations.

Do Your Homework

Even if you are willing to consult with a qualified herbalist,
and especially if you are not, you should do your homework
on alternative remedies before using them. This begins with
finding out everything you can about your condition and its
underlying causes. The source of your problem may be a cor-
rectable lifestyle issue such as chronic stress, a reaction to a
particular food, alcohol use, or a toxic item in your environment. If this is the case, no remedy will compensate for the
problem or yield a permanent result. Only after you have
eliminated these issues should you consider using an alternative remedy.

The next step is to consult with a qualified herbalist or, if
you are going to use remedies on your own, to learn as much
as possible about herbal medicine. There are many reference guides on both Western and Eastern herbs that describe
their basic properties and how they are used to treat various
health conditions. There is also information about herbs on

the Internet. Sales clerks in the supplement sections of natural food stores are often very knowledgeable about the uses of herbs.

When anyone recommends a remedy or an herb to you, be sure to check it out on your own before using it. Supplement sections of large natural food stores provide the computer database *Healthnotes Online*® free to their customers. This software program allows you to research and print information on a variety of herbs, remedies, and health conditions.

Read and compare manufacturers' labels to determine how remedies differ from one another. Note differences in quality and potency of the same remedy among different brands as well as differences in the amount and type of ingredients contained in the remedy.

Once you decide on an herb or remedy, you may want to shop around to get the best price. Natural food stores usually stock the greatest variety and highest quality of alternative remedies on the market, but you can sometimes find the same remedies online or by mail order at significantly lower prices.

Be Selective

Be selective about the remedies you choose to use because of their variances. For example, echinacea is available in many forms and dosages. If combined with goldenseal, it becomes an entirely different remedy than when used alone. Choose remedies with the freshest bioactive materials. Moisture, light, and air all have an adverse effect on the freshness of herbs. Make sure that herbs are organically grown, have not been sprayed with pesticides, herbicides, or other toxic materials, and contain no unusual substances such as pharmaceutical drugs.

Check the processing and standardization of remedies. Standardization means that a remedy is analyzed to verify the percentage content of the ingredients. It usually results in greater consistency and the assurance that you are actually getting the amounts of the herb that you need. Compare ingredients in formulas, and ask questions about how the differences will impact your treatment.

Safety should be a primary concern. Will the remedy have an effect on other medicines, what are the consequences if you take it longer than you should or exceed the recommended dosage, and does it contain any harmful ingredients? Some imported Chinese remedies were found to contain ingredients such as acetaminophen and low doses of arsenic, the latter of which can be extremely hazardous to your health. It is also not easy to find out what is contained in a remedy if the ingredients listed on the package happen to be in another language.

Pay attention to expiration dates listed on alternative remedy labels. Homeopathic medicines are effective for a very long time, but other remedies may lose their potency one to five years from the date of manufacture. Lot numbers also refer to the date of manufacture, but you must contact the manufacturer to find out what it is. Pay particular attention to expiration dates on mail-order remedies. Although mail-order remedies are competitively priced, they often expire sooner than the same remedies sold by retail stores because they sit on the shelf for a longer period of time.

Follow Instructions

There is a belief in conventional medicine that the strongest medicine is the best and shortest route to resolving a health condition. The reverse of this axiom is true in alternative medicine. In fact, the weakest strength of an herb or remedy is frequently the shortest route to healing. Homeopathic remedies are a good example of this phenomenon. *Alternative remedies do not become more effective the more you take them.* Always follow the manufacturer's directions for use, and never exceed the recommended dose listed on the label unless otherwise prescribed by a qualified herbalist. Taking too much of a remedy can not only be toxic but can also impede the body's natural immunity instead of enhancing it.

Find out how the alternative remedy is best administered. Some remedies should be taken with food, on an empty stomach, before meals, diluted in warm water, or at certain times or intervals of the day in order to be properly assimilated into the body. Sometimes, instructions for use are listed on the manufacturer label or package insert, but sometimes they are not. Instructions for use may also be found in herbal medicine guides and from qualified herbalists.

Pay Attention

Be aware of changes that occur when you take an alternative remedy, so you know how best to proceed in your treatment. In conventional medicine, we are used to relying on the expertise of doctors and the results of diagnostic tests in order to know if a medicine is working properly. This reliance devalues your own observations and experiences. In alternative medicine, your observations and experiences are held in higher regard, but assuming this responsibility requires some acclimatizing if you are not used to it.

Notice changes not only in your physical condition but also in your mental and spiritual condition as well.

Remember that alternative remedies affect a person on every level. Changes can be very subtle but nonetheless profound. Do not be discouraged if an alternative remedy does not provide immediate results. Remedies frequently take a long time to work and can continue to be effective even after you have discontinued their use. On the other hand, no change can also mean that you have not yet found the right remedy.

Take Frequent Breaks

Take frequent breaks from an alternative remedy to give your body a chance to rest and the remedy a chance to work. A remedy or herb taken on a short-term basis may be able to alleviate symptoms to the extent that you can then recognize and resolve the underlying causes that were previously obscured. Remedies support and enhance the body's own natural healing process, which is then stimulated and encouraged to act on its own when they are discontinued. If you do not break from a remedy, your body is not encouraged to act on its own and may become too dependant on the medicine.

We have a propensity in our culture to use medicine longer than we should, believing that the longer we take it, the more effective it will be. In alternative medicine, once again, the opposite is usually true.

Alternative remedies are intended to be used for limited periods of time and are usually more effective when applied in this manner. They should not be used on a long-term basis unless so prescribed and supervised by a qualified herbalist. Taking a remedy too long has the same effect as taking too much of it. It can have toxic consequences and interfere with the body's own natural ability to defend itself.

When to Stop Taking a Remedy

Stop taking an alternative remedy if it is clearly not helping you or is making your condition worse. You must keep in mind, however, that alternative interventions frequently result in a healing crisis in which symptoms become worse before getting better. When you use alternative remedies on your own, you must be able to tell the difference between a healing crisis and a bad outcome. This is another reason to pay close attention to any changes in your condition from taking an alternative remedy. If you can make this distinction, you can prevent an adverse reaction from turning into a more serious problem.

In the presence of an adverse reaction, you must be able to discern the difference between a bad outcome that is caused by the remedy and one that is caused by other factors in your life that have nothing to do with the remedy. Try eliminating possible factors one at a time. If an outside problem or upset resolves and the symptoms remain, the remedy may indeed be the cause of the adverse reaction. If you stop taking the remedy and the symptoms remain after a reasonable period of time, the outside problem may be the cause of it.

Keep Your Doctor Informed

Tell your medical doctor that you are taking an alternative remedy or herb, particularly if he is treating you for a serious health condition. Although studies show that most people do not do this, it is important for your health. Remedies can interact with conventional drugs in both positive and negative ways, and you do not want one medicine working against the other. For example, studies have found that the herb St. John's Wort makes several prescription medicines less effective, including drugs used to treat HIV infection, drugs to help prevent organ transplant rejection, birth control pills, and cholesterol-lowering medications.

If your conventional doctor disparages your use of alternative remedies, take the time to explain to him why using them is important to you and your health. If your doctor is unable to identify the interactive risks of medicines, encourage him to read more about them so you can engage in more mutually informed discussions. Sharing your positive alternative remedy experiences with your doctor will eventually lead to more support for their use. The more open you are in discussing them, the more open doctors will be in regarding them as a serious option in the treatment of health conditions.

Top 25 Alternative Remedies

There are several alternative remedies and herbs that address a wide range of minor health conditions and are easy to use on your own. Remedies and herbs, however, should not be prescribed without consideration for all the factors discussed in this chapter, especially in the presence of a serious health condition.

Many of the herbs in the list that follows may be combined with other herbs in compounded formulas to optimize their healing attributes and enhance their overall effectiveness. Western herbs are frequently combined with Eastern herbs, which collectively are considered to be more varied and thorough in addressing health imbalances.

The *Top 25 Alternative Remedies* to address general health complaints on your own are:

Homeopathic Remedies

1. **Arnica** (*Arnica montana*) is a homeopathic remedy available in both an external and internal preparation and used to treat bruises, dislocations, fractures, head injuries, joint, and muscle injuries. Topricin®, a topical cream that combines arnica with other homeopathic remedies, also addresses pain and inflammation issues.

2. **Oscillococcinum™** is a trademark homeopathic remedy taken internally and used to treat influenza. It is most effective if taken within 48 hours of the onset of flu symptoms.

Western Remedies

3. **Rescue Remedy™** is a trademark Bach flower essence combination remedy used to calm and stabilize the body in acutely stressful situations. **Five Flower Formula™** is the same flower essence combination made by another company.

4. **Tea tree oil** (*Melaleuca alternifolia*) is an essential oil derived from the leaves of an Australian tree. It is used as an antiseptic and disinfectant for a wide variety of conditions and has antibacterial, antifungal, and antiviral properties.

5. **Garlic** (*Allium sativum*) is one of the best known and most globally used culinary herbs with numerous health properties. Garlic lowers cholesterol, protects against heart disease, stimulates the immune system, and lowers blood pressure. Along with its cousin the onion, garlic is used for colds, flu, fevers, infections, blood pressure,

headaches, parasites, as an anticancer agent, and as a tonic for cardiovascular conditions. Garlic is available as a lozenge, pill, and in its raw, natural state.

6. **Ginger** (*Zingiber officinalis*) is a warming herbal stimulant and an anti-inflammatory root and is used to benefit digestion, elimination, and circulation. It is extremely effective when used to treat indigestion, motion sickness, and nausea. Ginger is eaten fresh or cooked in a tea. It is also used externally for inflamed or stiff joints.

7. **Peppermint** (*Mentha piperita*) is a popular remedy for digestive and eliminative conditions. As an antibacterial, peppermint is a common ingredient in various analgesics for external use. Peppermint essential oil is used topically to alleviate headaches.

8. **Echinachea** (*Echinacea angustifolia*) is a Native American plant whose root has powerful antibiotic, anti-inflammatory, and immunostimulation properties. It is a blood and lymphatic cleanser and is used to treat colds, flu, acute and chronic bacterial and viral infections, and many other conditions. Echinachea is used as a tea or an extract and is often combined with goldenseal or zinc. Externally it can be used to heal wounds.

9. **Aloe vera** (*Aloe vera*) is the gel extracted from the leaves of the aloe plant and is extremely effective in treating burns and rashes. It is also used to treat bug stings and acne. High levels of aloe vera in capsule form are used internally as a laxative as is the herb **Senna** *(Cassia angustifolia)*.

10. **Feverfew** (*Tanacetum parthenium*) is an herb whose leaves and flowers are used primarily to treat

headaches, particularly migraine headaches. This herb must be taken regularly for several weeks in order for it to be effective. Feverfew is also used for colds, flu, fevers, and digestive problems.

11. **Valerian** (*Valeriana officinalis*) is an herb whose root is used in tinctures, pills, and teas to sedate and calm the nervous system, alleviate emotional disturbances, and reduce pain. It is a relatively safe remedy for insomnia and is often found in combination with other effective herbal sedatives such as **Passion Flower** (*Passi flora incarnata*) and **Hops** (*Humulus lupus*). **Kava kava** (*Piper methysticum*) is another herb with anti-anxiety properties, but recent reports of liver problems from its use warrant extreme caution.

12. **Witch Hazel** (*Hamamelis virginiana*) is used as an astringent for all types of typical household injuries and to treat physical conditions such as diarrhea. It is most often found in the form of a distilled liquid and can be applied both internally and externally.

13. **Chamomile** (*Matricaria recutita*) flowers are commonly used to make a tea that aids digestion, acts as a mild sedative, and provides anti-inflammatory properties. Chamomile is used internally for various problems with the gastrointestinal tract. This versatile herb can also be used externally for other inflammatory conditions.

14. **Vitamin E** in liquid form is used topically to treat cuts and wounds and helps to prevent scarring. Taken internally, it is a powerful antioxidant known to retard aging and reduce hot flashes in menopausal women.

15. **Acidophilus** culture complexes are beneficial bacteria that maintain a healthy intestinal environment. They counteract pathogens and synthesize nutrients in the

intestines. Supplemental acidophilus, which must be stored in the refrigerator, helps constipation and replaces beneficial bacteria destroyed by conventional antibiotics.

16. **Essential oils** are used in aromatherapy and are antimicrobial on contact. **Camphor** is an essential oil known to strengthen immunity. **Roman chamomile** and **lavender** are essential oils known for their calming properties. **Peppermint** essential oil aids digestion and externally treats headaches. Select only pure essential oils whose fragrances are personally appealing to you.

17. **Digestive enzymes** aid digestion and indigestion. Enzymes like pancreatin and bromelain are anti-inflammatory if taken on an empty stomach. Digestive enzymes are made from ingredients like papaya and other natural ingredients and are available in capsules, gelcaps, and flavored, chewable tablets.

Eastern Remedies

18. **Pemenkanwan** and **Bi Yan Pian** are Chinese remedies that are available in pill form. They are known as patent medicines and are used to treat allergies and hay fever. **Nettle** (*Urtica dioica*), also known as Stinging Nettle, is the Western herb most commonly used to treat allergies and asthma.

19. **Gan Mao Ling** and **Yin Chiao** are Chinese remedies for colds and sore throats.

20. **Zhon Gan Ling** is a Chinese remedy used to treat symptoms of the flu and colds, including fever and chills.

21. **Ginseng** (men) and **Dong Quoi** (women) are the supreme Chinese herbs for revitalizing the body and

mind. There are many forms of ginseng—Korean, Siberian, and Chinese. Ginseng and dong quoi are believed to enhance overall energy, longevity, and sexual performance.

22. **Curing Pills** is a Chinese remedy used to aid most digestive problems, nausea, and diarrhea. It is a useful remedy to take with you when traveling to other countries.

23. **Tiger Balm™** is an aromatic Chinese analgesic effective for bruises and muscle aches.

Miscellaneous

24. **Medicinal Teas** are packaged in a variety of Western and Eastern herbal combinations to alleviate specific physical and mental conditions like colds, flu, PMS, and stress among many others. Herbal teas are naturally decaffeinated and come in loose form or tea bags. For example, Traditional Medicinals™ Breathe Easy is an herbal tea formula used for congestion. Chinese green tea, which is caffeinated and made from the *Camellia sinensis* plant, is known to offer a variety of health benefits. Tulsi tea is the Indian equivalent of green tea.

25. **Cold packs** and **moist hot packs** address acute inflammatory injuries and chronic musculoskeletal conditions respectively. Cold retards blood flow to the affected area while heat speeds it up. Use cold at the first sign of injury and use heat 48 hours after the injury occurs. Chronic conditions usually respond best to alternating cold and hot compresses.

Hot packs are usually cloth covered, filled with whole grains such as rice or buckwheat and aromatic herbs, and heated in a microwave oven. Cold packs are usually filled with dry ice that is activated when broken or a gel-like substance that is chilled in the freezer. Hot and cold packs are found at pharmacies, health food and herb stores, and from bodyworkers.

Herbal Travel Kit

Most of the remedies and herbs described above can be adapted into a convenient travel kit to address minor complaints when you are away from home. Many of them are also purchasable in convenient travel sizes. Remember to wrap remedies such as essential oils carefully and separately, so they do not leak into your travel case. Favorites for travel include:

1. **Arnica**—cream or gel for sore muscles

2. **Calendula**—cream or gel for skin irritations and cuts

3. **Aloe Vera**—cream or gel for skin burns and irritations

4. **Tiger Balm™**—salve for very sore muscles

5. **Digestive Aids**—chewable tablets for before or during meals

6. **Kava Kava or Valerian**—tablets or capsules for sleep

7. **Aconitum Napellus**—acute formula for sudden onset colds

8. **Oscillococcinum®**—sudden onset flu

9. **Lavender**—essential oil for relaxation

10. **Ginger**—tablets or tea bags for nausea

11. **Peppermint/Chamomile**—essential oil or teabags for headaches and fatigue

12. **Herbal lip balm and nonchemical sunscreen**—sun protection

13. **Natural eye drops** (i.e., Boiron Optique®)—irritated and tired eyes

SUMMARY & FURTHER READING

The Herbs of Life, Lesley Tierra, L.Ac., Herbalist

The Way of Herbs, Michael Tierra, L.Ac., O.M.D.

The Healing Power of Herbs, Michael Murray, N.D.

Healthy Healing, Linda Page, N.D., Ph.D.

Prescription for Nutritional Healing, James F. Balch, M.D. and Phyllis A. Balch, CNC

1. Consult with a qualified herbalist or other specialist in herbal medicine.

2. Do your homework on herbs and remedies, and shop around.

3. Be selective about the alternative remedies you choose because there is great variance in the quality of products.

4. Take alternative remedies according to packaged instructions or an herbalist's prescription, and never exceed the recommended dose.

5. Pay close attention to changes in your condition. Do not give up on an alternative remedy if there are not immediate results.

6. Take frequent breaks from using alternative remedies. They are generally not intended to be used continuously, for an extended period of time, or indefinitely.

7. Stop taking an alternative remedy in the event of an adverse reaction, and consult with a qualified herbalist. Keep in mind that remedies and herbs can cause a healing crisis in which symptoms sometimes become worse before improving. Consult with your medical doctor about possible reactions with conventional drugs.

8. Keep your health care providers informed about all drugs, remedies, and herbs you are taking, especially if you are being treated for a serious health condition.

Herbal/Plant Therapy Organizations

Herb Research Foundation (303) 449–2265

American Botanical Council (512) 926–4900

American Herbalists Guild (770) 751–6021

World Wide Essence Society (978) 369–8454

American Association of Naturopathic Physicians
(866) 538–2267

American Horticulture Therapy Association
(800) 634–1603

CHAPTER 5

Six Steps to Using Alternative Medicine

Please note: *There is no guarantee of illness prevention or healing from any medicine. The alternative medicine suggestions in this chapter are intended to be adjunctive and not a substitute for conventional medicine. Consult your medical doctor before beginning any alternative medicine treatment program or lifestyle change. Remember to make changes safely and gradually.*

■ STEP ONE—**Assess Your Lifestyle**—*A Precondition to Alternative Medicine Treatment*

    1. Nutrition
    2. Exercise
    3. Rest & Relaxation
    4. Environment

■ STEP TWO—**Balance Your Space**—*"External Energy Work"*

Consult with an external energetic specialist about environmental balance. Examples are:

    1. Feng Shui
    2. Vastu Shastra

■ STEP THREE—**Balance Your Energy**—*"Internal Energy Work"*
Choose a comprehensive alternative medicine system
to incorporate into your healing program. Examples are:

    1. Chinese medicine
    2. Homeopathy
    3. Ayurveda

■ STEP FOUR—**Balance Your Mind**—*"Mind Work"*
Choose appropriate mindwork tools to incorporate into
your healing program. Examples are:

    1. Immune-Building Characteristics
    2. Healing Attitude
    3. Hypnosis & Guided Imagery
    4. Regression Therapy
    5. Healing Connections
    6. Humor

■ STEP FIVE—**Balance Your Body**—*"Body Work"*
Choose appropriate bodywork therapies to incorporate
into your healing program. Examples are:

    1. Massage Therapy
    2. Craniosacral Therapy
    3. Feldenkrais Method
    4. Polarity Therapy
    5. Medical Qigong

■ STEP SIX—**Prevent Future Imbalance**—*"Soul Work"*
Initiate the regular practice of an inward discipline.
Examples are:

    1. Meditation
    2. Yoga
    3. Qigong
    4. Tai Chi

All health care is based on the restoration of harmony and balance to the body, mind, and spirit. There are many paths to healing and many routes to arriving on the same path. The plan that follows divides alternative medicine treatment into six steps: lifestyle factors, the balance of external energy, the balance of internal energy, our thought processes, the release of physical restriction and limitation, and protection from future imbalance and disharmony. These six steps represent a type of dynamic mobile of health. The imbalance of any one factor disrupts the balance of all other factors in this treatment approach to alternative medicine.

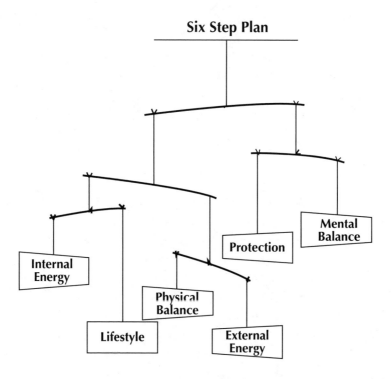

Fig. 2. Mobile of Health

Categories of Alternative Medicine

There are many different kinds of alternative medicine. *Comprehensive systems* of alternative medicine such as Chinese medicine utilize a variety of approaches and methods. *Subsystems* of alternative medicine represent a particular approach or modality like nutrition, herbology, and bodywork. Subsystems or modalities can exist within or outside of comprehensive alternative systems. Within alternative systems and modalities, there are *techniques, therapies, methods,* and *interventions.*

The National Center for Complementary and Alternative Medicine groups alternative medicine into five categories: alternative medicine systems, mind-body interventions, biologically based therapies, manipulative or body-based methods, and energy therapies. It is important, however, to remember that any responsible alternative practice is energetic in nature, impacts the mind, and is based in nature.

The Steps

The six-step plan provides a framework or formula for using any alternative practice. The goal of alternative medicine is to achieve overall balance by addressing body, mind, and spirit as one. These aspects of health are treated at one time because it is impossible to separate them. In this view, if you treat the body, mind and spirit are also affected. For the purpose of simplicity, however, the steps in this treatment approach are labeled with a specific focus even though they clearly overlap one another.

Examples of established alternative practices are briefly described to define and clarify each step. There are hundreds more alternative practices than are listed in the six-step plan.

The purpose of the plan is not to provide you with a list of all alternative practices or to determine which practices you should use. It is to provide you with an understandable framework for using alternative medicine from which you can choose the practice that is right for you. Remember that a practice that is right for one person may not be right for another. Once a practice is chosen, you must learn as much about it as possible from reliable resources, some of which are listed at the beginning of each step.

Except for *Steps One* and *Two*, the remaining steps are not arranged in any order of importance. In fact, a multifaceted approach that utilizes a combination of treatment steps is preferable, if you can afford to engage in more than one practice at a time. Remember that it is better to address one step completely than several steps partially or inadequately. You should feel no pressure to perform every step in the plan, and you should take on only what you feel you can handle comfortably.

If you participate in more than one practice at one time, do not schedule more than one treatment in a day because combining treatments on the same day can alter their effectiveness. Some of the steps may also not apply to your particular condition or situation.

Costs of Alternative Medicine

The average rates for service for alternative treatment range from $50-$150, depending on the experience and skill of the practitioner and excluding initial consultations, which are usually more costly because they require more time than follow-up appointments. Private psychotherapy services fall into this range, depending on the license held by the therapist. Instruction for inward disciplines such as yoga is usually $5-$15 per class or by donation for disciplines such as meditation.

Many alternative practitioners offer a sliding fee scale or, in the case of bodywork, a discount for a series of treatments. Fees for alternative medicine are frequently negotiable, particularly if insurance does not cover it. If the service is a covered expense and you still want to pay in cash, always ask for a cash discount.

Keys to Using Alternative Medicine

Taking responsibility for your health is the basis for any successful treatment approach and can take many forms. A *positive practitioner-consumer relationship* and *simplifying your lifestyle* as much as possible are precursors to the creation of a healing environment, as is *emotional support* from family or friends. You should *eliminate unhealthy lifestyle habits* that impede the ability of the medicine to work properly. To ensure the safe use of alternative methods, it is important to *make changes gradually*. Although breathwork is an important lifestyle change discussed in *Step One*, it is an integral part of almost every alternative practice. The Latin word for breath also means spirit, and the *use of the breath* is an important key to unlocking the door to many levels of healing.

STEP ONE
Assess Your Lifestyle

A Precondition to Alternative Medicine Treatment

SUMMARY & FURTHER READING

1. **Nutrition**—Eat a low-saturated fat, complex carbohydrate diet.

   Transition to Vegetarianism, Rudolph Ballantine

   Are You Confused?, Paava Airola

2. **Exercise**—Engage in regular physical activity.

3. **Rest & Relaxation**—Take regular quiet time.
   Learn to use the breath.
   Improve sleeping habits.

4. **Environment**—Reduce or remove toxins from your space.

   The Cure for All Disease, Hulda Regehr Clark Ph.D., N.D.

   Chemical Deception, The Toxic Threat to Health and Environment, Marc Lappe

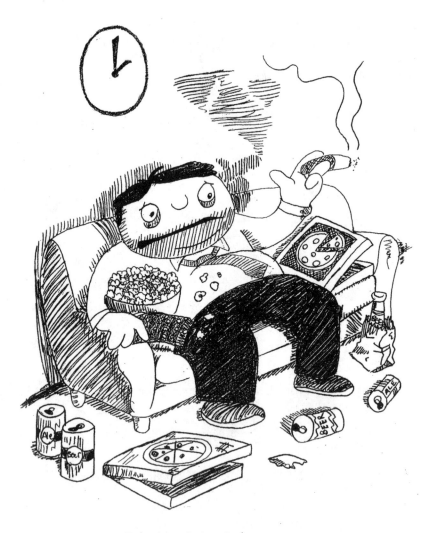

"I don't get it, I go in for accupuncture
every week and *still* feel lousy!"

In many ways, technology has made our lives more complicated instead of simplifying them. It is responsible for the mass production of food deficient in nutritional value from processing and treated with pesticides, herbicides, and other chemicals; a constant barrage of overstimulating images and information from a mass media; modern conveniences that have reduced physical activity to the point at which we are overly sedentary and must compensate with planned physical exercise; more efficient yet highly toxic products for the household; and many sources of environmental pollution.

In the long run, bigger, more, and faster have not proven to be better. As a society, we are just beginning to come to terms with the fact that growth does not always equal progress. Positive growth requires common sense and good judgment. In many respects, we have lost the ability to tell the difference between what is better for us and what is not, allowing commercial interests to dictate change. Our lives are certainly more convenient, but convenience definitely comes at a price!

It is old news that lifestyle habits impact health. Study after study confirms it. Good nutrition, regular exercise, adequate rest, and a toxic-free environment are all important factors in any health program, and no discussion of alternative medicine would be complete without their consideration.

Although we have heard it all before, we still tend to dismiss or ignore unhealthy lifestyle habits if we think there is an alternative to addressing them. Most people would rather take a pill to correct high blood pressure than alter their diet or initiate a regular exercise program. The problem with this thinking is that *there really is no substitute for healthy lifestyle habits in order to be and to stay well.* This includes alternative medicine.

The lifestyle issues outlined in this step are a precondition to all subsequent steps in the six-step plan. They must be operational in some form before any alternative treatment is initiated or the effectiveness of the treatment will be compromised. Good nutrition, regular exercise, adequate rest, and a toxic-free environment are all essential and basic components of health.

Other steps in the six-step plan address lifestyle issues such as the development of social connections in *Step Four* and the practice of an inward discipline in *Step Six*, which can be regarded as both an exercise and a means to relax.

NUTRITION
"Eat Right!"

After becoming a modified vegetarian more than three decades ago, I was the object of great ridicule by my friends. My own father used to point to my health food and say, "no preservatives, no additives, no good!" It was a time when nutrition experts widely disagreed on the best food lifestyle, medical doctors routinely maligned the notion that diet impacts health, and fad diets ruled the marketplace. No one is laughing anymore. My friends now compete with each other to have the healthiest lifestyles, and medical doctors have finally acknowledged the health benefits of both food and nutritional supplements.

We know more than we ever did before about what constitutes a healthy diet. We are aware of the potential healing power of many foods and the fact that poor nutrition is a leading cause of death and disease in the world. Despite all this information and according a recent survey conducted by the Centers for Disease Control and Prevention (CDC), almost one-third of the population is obese (one in five adults) and almost two-thirds of the population is overweight, which represents a steady increase during the past two decades.

Despite provocative new theories on what we should consume and avoid, including eating according to your blood type and carbohydrate addiction, the majority of nutrition experts still agree that a *low-saturated fat, low-protein, complex carbohydrate diet that is also low in cholesterol, refined, processed, and artificial foods is the most nutritionally beneficial lifestyle.* Optimum nutritional intake is generally defined as 50–70% carbohydrates, 10–20% protein, and 15–30% fat, with protein and fat less than one-half the total food consumption. Carbohydrates should be complex (whole grains, etc.) and fats should be essential (omega fatty acids, etc.).

This is the point at which it gets confusing to many people because there are fats that are actually good for you and carbohydrates that are not. But this is nothing new. The importance of discriminating among fats and carbohydrates to promote health and achieve permanent weight loss has been in the public health domain for decades, despite what you may have recently heard in the media.

Challengers of the low-saturated fat diet claim that carbohydrates make us fatter and more prone to disease. However, the only outcome of low-carbohydrate diets so far observed by scientists is short-term weight loss, and only a small percentage of the population is actually carbohydrate-sensitive. All nutrition camps do agree that you should try to consume complex carbohydrates rather than ones that are highly refined or processed such as white sugar, white flour, and white rice.

Disagreement still exists about optimum protein level, yet evidence shows that the countries with low rates of disease and the greatest longevity eat low protein diets. There is no evidence to show that high protein diets improve your health long term, but there is some evidence that they can cause liver and kidney problems. If these diets are high in saturated fat, they can also contribute to heart disease.

What seems most clear when it comes to nutrition is that individual requirements and moderation should always dictate the optimum food lifestyle.

Although we are still more focused on our weight than our health, for many people, the only way to achieve the latter is through permanent, sensible weight loss. *This can only be achieved by eating less, eating better, and exercising more.* There is simply no shortcut to this process and no miracle theory or program, as yet undiscovered, which will allow you to avoid performing these three tasks.

For me, achieving health involved a year-long transition from the typical American diet to a modified vegetarian one, including a small amount of seafood and dairy. There are now many forms of vegetarianism: some vegetarians consume eggs (ovo) or dairy (lacto) and vegans (pronounced vēēgan) avoid intake of all animal products including dairy, eggs, and honey.

There are some common misconceptions about vegetarians. All vegetarians do not eat tofu and huge amounts of dairy to compensate for the lack of meat, and contrary to what many restaurants chefs think (given the size of most vegetarian entrees), they are not on diets! In fact, vegetarians must actually consume more volume than meat-eaters in order to feel similarly satiated.

Whatever nutritional lifestyle you chose, make changes to your diet slowly and make sure that the foods you consume are healthy and nutritious. It takes a long time to change your eating habits and your overall attitude about food, but an amazing thing happens when you do—the longer you eat this way, the more you *want* to eat this way. A common sense list of *10 Nutritional Do's includes:*

1. Eat the good fats, and avoid the bad ones.

2. Eat less processed, refined, and artificial food.

3. Eat low glycemic-load complex carbohydrates.

4. Drink more water.

5. Simplify what you eat.

6. Eat smaller, frequent meals.

7. Avoid smoking and alcohol.

8. Read food labels.

9. Take nutritional supplements.

10. Eat in moderation.

Good Fats & Bad Fats

All fats are not created equal. Some fats are necessary for optimum health, but other fats are harmful. The type of fat you eat is far more important than the amount of fat you eat. Scientific research has shown that there are many health risks associated with the consumption of a high animal fat diet that is also high in saturated fat and cholesterol.

Consumption of saturated fat is linked to many diseases and health conditions including heart and kidney disease, breast and prostate cancer, fatigue, and intestinal, digestive, and gynecological disorders. Most experts agree that your intake of saturated fat should be reduced for these reasons. Believe it or not, a high animal fat diet is also associated with body odor, which we have learned to conceal through the use of underarm deodorants, perfumes, and colognes.

Meat, poultry, fish, eggs, and dairy products all contain saturated fat. Saturated fat is also found in coconuts, palm oil, chocolate, vegetable shortening, hydrogenated oils such as margarine, and partially hydrogenated oils. In order to reduce your intake of saturated fat, limit your intake of high-fat meats and dairy products as much as possible.

Butter, which is high in saturated fat, is less harmful for you than margarine. This is true even if the margarine is low in cholesterol and fat because margarine contains potentially harmful transfatty acids. Trans fat is directly associated with heart disease, decreasing good cholesterol (HDL) and boosting bad cholesterol (LDL). The majority of trans fat comes from hydrogenation, which is the process of turning vegetable oil into a product that remains solid at room temperature like margarine or shortening.

Trans fat is also found in partially hydrogenated oils used in commercially baked products and fast foods, particularly fried foods. Fried foods have also been found to contain the chemical acrylamide, which causes cancer. Oils heated to high temperatures are not only believed to be harmful for you, but overcooking also alters and destroys valuable nutrients in food. Try to eliminate trans fat from your diet because no amount of it is good for you.

Intake of vegetable oils that are high in unsaturated or polyunsaturated fat (corn, safflower, soy, sesame, and sunflower) should also be reduced or avoided. Although they provide essential fatty acids, polyunsaturated fat lowers both good and bad cholesterol and is believed to possess cancer-causing agents.

Avoid the artificial fat substitutes that are used to make fat-free foods. It is better for you to eat a reduced-fat food than one made with an artificial fat substitute. To reduce fat in baking, replace oil and butter with fruits like mashed banana and unsweetened applesauce and use egg whites rather than whole eggs. Remember that fat-free does not mean calorie-free.

Select vegetable oils that are expeller-pressed, unrefined, organic, and high in monounsaturated fat, which lowers only bad cholesterol. Monounsaturated fat is found in olive, canola, peanut, and avocado oils. Extra virgin olive oil has many health benefits and is the ideal oil to use in cooking.

Although most polyunsaturated fat is not good for you, there is a category of polyunsaturated fat termed omega–3 fatty acids that falls outside those parameters. Oily fish such as salmon, sardines, and mackerel contains high levels of omega–3 fatty acids. Omega–3 fatty acids are also found in flaxseed oil and, to a lesser degree, in walnut, black currant, soy, and canola oils. These essential fatty acids (EFA) are fuel that the body needs in order to be healthy and are both anti-inflammatory and heart-protective. These are the good fats.

Although fish contains beneficial omega–3 fats, large fish such as shark, swordfish, king mackerel, tilefish, and tuna contain high levels of methylmercury. The Food and Drug Administration (FDA) recommends that pregnant women avoid eating these fish because methylmercury is a pollutant that can cause damage to the fetus. A recent study also suggested that the consumption of fish with a high mercury content may also increase the risk of heart attack, negating the heart-protective benefits of omega–3 fats. Remember that the larger the fish, the higher the potential mercury content.

Soybean products have become very popular among the health-conscious, particularly as a substitution for meat and dairy. The proponents of soy claim that it has many health benefits, including reducing the risk for heart disease, breast and prostate cancer, and menopausal symptoms. Only fermented soy products such as tempeh, miso, and tamari are actually beneficial, especially when combined with other protein-rich foods such as those consumed in the Orient.

Unfermented soy products are extremely difficult to digest and prevent the absorption of important minerals, which can affect the functioning of the brain and nervous system. The fermentation process breaks down the carbohydrates, making them more digestible, and permits mineral absorption. Consumption of a high soy diet, as a replacement for meat and dairy, is not safe and may actually increase the risk for disease instead of reducing it.

Increase your consumption of organic fresh vegetables, fresh fruits, whole grains, and legumes, which naturally contain complete protein, a high vitamin and mineral content, fiber, and essential fats. These foods help prevent heart disease, diabetes, and certain cancers. Plant foods like nuts, seeds, avocados, soybeans, and olives are nutritious in the proper form and amount but have a natural high fat content. If you are on a fat-restricted diet, you may want to limit your intake of these foods.

Organic Food

The word "organic" is used frequently and means different things to different people. Organic food is generally supposed to be unprocessed and free of synthetic pesticides, herbicides, fungicides, and chemical fertilizers. In the past, food producers were allowed to claim that their products were organic whether they were or not. Now that sales of organic foods has reached $6 billion per year, the U.S. Department of Agriculture published federal standards for organic food, which became effective October 21, 2002.

According to these standards, foods labeled organic must contain 95% organically produced ingredients. In addition to the conditions cited above, organic foods must also be free of irradiation, biotechnology, and sewage sludge, and meats must be free of antibiotics. Foods that qualify receive a "USDA Organic" stamp from the federal government. Products that state they are "made with organic ingredients" must be at least 70% organic but are ineligible for the USDA stamp. Remember that organic meat and produce spoil quicker than nonorganic versions because they are free of chemicals, so you must shop for them more frequently.

The phrase "all natural" is only a marketing term. It is not regulated and can mean anything or nothing.

Good Carbohydrates & Bad Carbohydrates

All carbohydrates are not created equal. There are carbohydrates that are good for you and those that are not. Complex carbohydrates are found in vegetables, fruits, and whole grains and have more vitamins, minerals, and fiber than simple carbohydrates, which are found in most sugars. Complex carbohydrates are also low in saturated fat. Unless you are starving yourself or you are overeating carbohydrates to compensate for a low-fat diet, carbohydrate cravings usually result from being overweight or hormonal.

Once ingested, carbohydrates are broken down into sugar. The amount of sugar and the speed of its release determine its glycemic index. The glycemic index and grams contained in each serving determine the glycemic load or the actual amount of carbohydrate in a serving of food. Low glycemic-load carbohydrates are preferable to high glycemic ones, particularly if you are carbohydrate-sensitive, because they take longer to digest and raise blood sugar levels more gradually. This allows the blood sugar in your body to stay at a consistent level for normal brain functioning, and you feel less hungry over the same period of time. For example, apples and asparagus convert to glucose slower than fruit juice or potatoes.

In general, the whiter, lighter, and spongier the food, the worse it is for you; the darker and denser the food, the better it is for you. *The three biggest, culinary culprits for wrecking havoc with our health are white sugar, white flour, and table salt.* White sugar and white flour are often characterized as "empty calories" because they are caloric but possess no nutritional value whatsoever.

We use white flour in everything from breads to pasta to sauces. Replace refined flours with whole grain or unrefined versions as much as possible. There are also whole grain pastry flours for making desserts or sweets. The blandness of white flour pales by comparison to flavorful whole grain versions. Sometimes, there is no difference in taste, and when there is, it is usually improved. The refinement process for any food involves the removal of valuable nutrients and fiber. Some experts believe that refined flour products are the actual cause of carbohydrate sensitivity.

Sweets are a comfort food, and since comfort is in short supply, it should be no surprise that ours is a sugar-addicted society. According to the U.S. Department of Agriculture, the average person consumes an astonishing 150 lbs. of sweeteners every year. Consumption of sweets is dangerous for certain health conditions such as diabetes and hypoglycemia, and high amounts of refined sugar deplete mental and physical energy by causing extreme fluctuations in blood sugar levels. Complex carbohydrates in foods such as starchy vegetables, legumes, whole grains, and fresh fruit not only satisfy the craving for sweets but also increase serotonin levels and improve mood.

Avoid white sugar or other sweeteners in processed foods, and avoid artificial sweeteners completely. Sodium saccharine was shown to cause cancer, and aspartame has been linked to brain cancer and other health problems. Remember that fat-free does not mean sugar free. In fact, additional sugar is often added to these products to compensate for the lack of fat.

If you cannot give up sweets completely, try making them at home, replacing refined sugar with moderate amounts of natural sweeteners, such as fruit juice concentrate (liquid or crystals), granulated cane juice, rice syrup, unfiltered honey, maple syrup, barley malt, and stevia herb extract. Desserts that are sugar-free are usually indistinguishable in taste from those made with refined sugar. There are several dessert cookbooks that use natural sweeteners in recipes in place of refined sugar. You can also purchase sweets made with natural sweeteners at natural food stores.

To recap, you should avoid white carbohydrates and the products made with them such as breads, pastas, and rice. But it is equally important to consume an adequate amount of healthy carbohydrates to avoid carbohydrate deficiency, which can cause as many health problems as carbohydrate addiction. Whole grains products, beans, and vegetables like winter squash, eggplant, and sweet potatoes should be an essential part of any balanced nutritional program.

Table Salt

Ours is also a salt-addicted society, in great part because heavily processed and overcooked food has little or no flavor and complexity, so we compensate for their absence with an excessive amount of table salt. We also use it as a preservative to extend the shelf life of mass produced food products. Table salt contains high amounts of sodium chloride, much more than the body needs. Although salt regulates water balance and controls nerve function, an excess of it puts strain on the heart and kidneys and raises blood pressure, also contributing to edema and stomach cancer. Most foods contain a sufficient amount of natural salt to satisfy daily requirements.

Reduce the amount of table salt you add to your meals, and begin to season food with fresh or dried herbs. Herbs taste better and are more nutritious for you. There are a number of salt-free seasoning products on the market that contain a combination of dried herbs. If you need to use salt, use natural sea salt, which is available at natural food stores. Once you begin to eat more fresh, unprocessed foods, the need for heavy seasonings will naturally dissipate.

Drink More Water

Approximately 60% of our body weight is water, and adequate intake of water facilitates nearly every bodily process including circulation, elimination, digestion, and temperature control. (Drinking water before and after a meal, rather than during it, also aids digestion.) Some experts believe that chronic dehydration is a contributing factor, if not an outright cause, of most health problems, including arthritis, allergies, asthma, overweight, high blood pressure, certain degenerative diseases, and emotional issues. This widespread dietary inadequacy is one very few people take seriously or feel compelled to correct.

The fact is that most of us do not consume enough water and are accustomed to replacing it with every kind of manufactured beverage imaginable. What plain, ole water does for you cannot be replaced with any flavored beverage. *If you can make only one change to your diet, drinking more water is the one change you should make.* Drinking water regularly will also eliminate the lack of it as a factor in serious health problems.

Find out what works for you—cold or room temperature, with lemon or lime. Get a refillable bottle to carry with you, so you can sip water throughout the day. Tap water is not what it used to be, so drink only pure bottled water that is free of chemicals and harmful bacteria. You know what they say—eight glasses a day!

Simplify Your Diet

Our society promotes the notion that variety is the spice of life; however, the healthiest countries in the world eat the same foods over and over again. A simplified diet does not promote boredom but consistency and health. It is not necessary to vary the food that you eat if you accept this premise. It is also easier to make changes to your diet if you eat simply. The simplest meals are the ones you make yourself, which is the only way for you to completely control what you consume. This is more difficult to accomplish if you eat a lot of convenience or restaurant food.

Eat Smaller, Frequent Meals

Consume smaller, more frequent meals during the course of a day rather than the three large traditional ones, particularly if you are carbohydrate-sensitive. Frequent meals help maintain proper blood sugar levels, increasing physical and mental energy and functioning. If you miss a meal and feel sluggish, your body often craves something sweet, but it is really craving glucose to the brain. If this happens, try eating a whole grain cracker or a piece of fresh fruit rather than a highly processed or sugared food. The former provides a more lasting release of glucose to the brain and satisfies the craving for sweets.

In general, protein gives you energy, which is why its consumption is recommended early in the day, and carbohydrates tend to slow you down, which is why their consumption is preferable in the evening.

Avoid Smoking & Alcohol

Smoking is a major cause of disease, including cancer and premature aging. Excessive alcohol consumption damages the nervous system and liver. What more needs to be said than this?

Read Food Labels

If you are serious about changing your eating habits, begin to check the ingredients on food labels. You may be surprised to learn what you have been putting into your body without knowing it. A good rule of thumb to follow is if you cannot pronounce it, you should not consume it. In this case, what you do not know *can* hurt you!

You should also check ingredients of products you purchase at natural food stores because not every product there is good for you. Natural food stores have changed dramatically over the past two decades. No longer the hippie stores of the 1960s, they have become the yuppie stores of the new century, catering to a much wider audience and trying to be all things to all people. Although health food used to represent the alternative to the typical American diet, there are more meat, dairy, and sugar products in natural food stores than ever before, particularly the larger ones such as Whole Foods and Wild Oats.

Please note that most conventional supermarkets in major metropolitan areas offer health food sections but do not provide the personal service typical of natural food stores.

Nutritional Supplements

Not long ago, medical doctors claimed vitamin and mineral supplements were superfluous in the presence of a proper diet and balanced nutrition. These doctors never bothered to consider that the food available to most of us is overprocessed, preserved with unhealthy chemicals, and adversely affected by environmental pollution. Now, science has shown that supplemental vitamins and minerals not only improve immunity and deter disease but also retard the aging process. Supplements are more necessary to health than ever before.

Nutritional supplements, which some people now term "nutraceuticals" as opposed to "pharmaceuticals", provide many vital health functions. Not only do they enhance immune response and protect against infection, but antioxidants like vitamin E prevent damage to cells; B vitamins aid enzyme function; and calcium builds and maintains bones, lowers blood pressure, and prevents colon cancer.

Nutritional supplements are available in many forms—tablets, gelcaps, powders, and liquids. Learn to read ingredient labels on nutritional supplements so you know what you are getting and how to use them. *Percent Daily Value (DV)* indicates the amount of the nutrient recommended by the Food and Drug Administration (FDA) that is in one serving. *Serving size* tells you the amount you must consume in order to get the *Percent Daily Value*. Scientific units of supplements are represented by *International Units (IU)*, a global standard for measuring supplements; *milligrams (mg)*; and *micrograms (mcg)*—one milligram equaling 1,000 micrograms.

The expiration date tells you when the potency of a supplement will be lost, affecting the *Percent Daily Value*. The lot number tells you the time and place of production.

Suggested use indicates dosage and storage information. *Warnings* usually refer to possible adverse effects if you are taking prescription medications, are pregnant, or have allergies. They may also alert you to broken or missing seals or caps of supplements, which should be returned to the place of purchase for an exchange or a refund.

The most reliable nutritional supplements are still found at reputable stores that specialize in natural foods or herbs. Large natural food stores also manufacture their own line of nutritional supplements. Solgar, Country Life, Rainbow Light, and Source Naturals are among the many reliable supplement manufacturers. Brand name supplements are available through mail-order suppliers like iHerb, The Vitamin Shoppe, and Nutrition Warehouse and on the Internet at sometimes greatly reduced prices.

It pays to shop around for nutritional supplements because prices for them can vary anywhere from 20% to 40%. Alternative practitioners sometimes sell nutritional supplements directly to their clients. If they engage in this practice, they should never charge you more than their actual cost for them.

Recent claims have been made that supplements in liquid form provide increased absorption over tablets or powders. There are advantages and disadvantages to liquids. Liquids are easier to swallow than pills or tablets and get into your system quickly because there is nothing to dissolve, but some vitamins spoil easily in liquid form. Gelcaps are easier to swallow and more assimilable than pills or tablets.

If you are unaccustomed to taking high-potency supplements, you need to build up to the recommended doses gradually. When dealing with illness, supplements in any form are best customized to your specific needs by a qualified alternative practitioner or nutritional specialist.

EXERCISE
"Move!"

You must move and breathe in some form of regular physical exercise in order to be well. Exercise is both preventive and curative and has many physiological benefits, including strength, endurance, flexibility, and vitality. Regular exercise increases longevity and reduces the risk for many health conditions including heart disease, cancer, diabetes, high blood pressure, depression, osteoporosis, and premature aging. A recent study demonstrated that a lack of exercise has a dramatic effect on longevity, one expert claiming that it is worse for your health than either smoking or obesity.

Remember that physical exercise only makes you physically fit. For total health, you must also engage in activities that promote mental and spiritual fitness, which are discussed in *Steps Four* and *Six*.

There are two factors to consider in choosing a physical exercise: you enjoy performing it and can do so with a reasonable degree of regularity.

Enjoyment

Exercise involves any physical activity that you enjoy performing and allows you to move, exercise your heart, and stretch your muscles. Exercise does not have to be a sport, an organized activity, or take place in a health club in order to provide health benefits. There is an endless array of choices for physical exercise, which range from those that have been around awhile such as running, cycling, swimming, weight lifting, boxing, climbing, riding, and brisk walking to new and rediscovered ones such as Pilates, spinning, and Tai Bo.

Contemplative disciplines such as yoga, *tai chi*, and *qigong* were designed to address not only physical fitness but also mental and spiritual health and well-being. These disciplines help focus the attention and free the mind and can be very relaxing. Try to incorporate a contemplative discipline into your health program at least once per week. The ideal fitness program includes cardiovascular or aerobic, weight-bearing, and stretching exercises. The bottom line is that you will not exercise if you do not enjoy doing it, so find an exercise that appeals to you.

Regularity

You must exercise on a regular basis in order to receive health benefits. Joining a fitness club or class, finding an exercise buddy, and picking a specific time of the day to exercise will help you do this. Some people need to exercise in the morning; others prefer the evening after work. Like dietary change, the longer you exercise, the more you will want to exercise. Regular exercise improves sleep, mood, stamina, circulation, self-esteem, and general well-being.

Recommendations are constantly being updated on the amount of exercise you need to promote health. The most recent study recommends at least one hour of moderate physical activity daily, twice the amount of time recommended by the U.S. Surgeon General in 1996. Do not let this discourage you. Any exercise you do is better than doing nothing, but you should try to exercise at least 30 minutes four to five times every week to receive health benefits.

REST & RELAXATION
"Slow Down!"

We have become locked into the bizarre notion that constant busyness is always good, which comes from living in an industrialized and highly urbanized society. Being occupied with work or a task is an asset when you need to get your mind off something and channel your efforts toward a productive cause or goal. But chronic busyness without adequate restoration creates stress, and chronic stress contributes to a whole range of health problems, both major and minor.

Eighty-five percent of illness has been attributed to emotional stress. Stress increases the likelihood of disease and has been linked to more health conditions than any other cause, including heart disease, autoimmunity, high blood pressure, all forms of pain, and sleeping disorders. Science has shown that the stress response interrupts several bodily functions, including the suppression of the immune system. Although it is known through studies that chronic stress impairs memory and damages neurons in the brain, a recent Israeli study demonstrated a connection between acute stress and actual brain damage.

Stress is defined as physical or mental tension or strain. There is acute stress, which normally resolves itself on its own, and chronic stress, which requires some form of self-management and personal or environmental adjustment. Although we differ in many ways, stress is probably the one health circumstance or condition that most of us share in common.

We deal with all types of environmental stressors every day—rising costs, traffic congestion, long lines, building construction, automated telephone menus, rude people, and the mass media, all of which overstimulate our central nervous systems and affect our overall health. Service industries no longer serve, companies avoid responsibility, and we are constantly bombarded with messages that pressure us to "buy, buy, buy."

How you handle ordinary stress determines, in great part, the extent to which it impacts your health. For example, you can have very healthy lifestyle habits but poor health if you are unable to handle everyday stress comfortably. On the other hand, you can have unhealthy lifestyle habits but good health if you are able to manage everyday stress easily. Another axiom is that the greater the stress, the more difficult it is to take the time to relax and alleviate it.

Moving from the city to the country, the current trend of stressed-out urbanites, will not automatically eliminate stress in your life because there is stress in the environment and stress of your own creation. You can change your environment but continue to be impacted by self-induced stress. You must simplify your life in order to reduce stress, facilitate relaxation, and stay healthy, and you can do this wherever you live.

Complicated lifestyles are a choice, not a necessity or obligation. Even if you eliminate stress of your own creation, however, you will still have to deal with a certain amount of environmental stress as an inexorable reality of living in a hectic world.

Stress management has become an integral part of developing healthy lifestyle habits, like washing your face or brushing your teeth. The value of rest and relaxation during illness cannot be overemphasized. It is during these times that you will need all of your resources for getting well, but they will not be available to you if you are stressed out.

Rest and relaxation involve periodic quiet time, using the breath, and restful sleep.

Regular Quiet Time

It is impossible to ameliorate the effects of daily stress without engaging in some form of regular relaxation. The cocktail hour is no longer considered an ideal way to unwind. In order to properly learn to relax, we must get over our discomfort with silence and the self-reflection that naturally arises from it.

The best way to relax and rejuvenate yourself is to *simplify the space around you* and *surround yourself with silence*. Allow yourself a moment of silence every day to think about nothing—even if it is only for five minutes, and sit quietly without interruption.

Lose yourself in nature or find a room where you can rest undisturbed, unplugging the telephone and turning off the volume on the answering machine. Allow your mind to wander, and imagine yourself disappearing in the light and shadows of the space. Be and do absolutely nothing. Give your body, mind, and psyche a genuine vacation from the stresses of everyday life because you deserve it.

Quiet time replenishes the soul, particularly if you engage in practices such as yoga or meditation. If doing nothing is difficult for you in the beginning, take hot baths, go for long walks, or listen to relaxation tapes to get yourself accustomed to the solitary experience. Self-hypnosis is also an excellent tool for relaxation, which you can learn from a hypnotist or on your own from the many available guides on the topic.

Progressive relaxation training (PRT) is another tool you can use to unwind. Progressive relaxation involves alternately tensing and relaxing groups of muscles and is performed sitting or lying down. Start at one end of your body, tense a body part, and release it for twice the amount of time that you tensed it. Repeat this process for each body part throughout the body (face, neck, shoulders, etc.).

Many people erroneously believe that watching television, reading, and playing with children is relaxing, but these activities are actually more stimulating than restorative. Be highly selective about the amount and source of news and entertainment that you absorb in a day. News and entertainment with a focus on negativity or violence are not only physiologically stimulating but also psychologically distressing and can affect both waking and sleeping states. This is especially true in the broadcast media, which has become both assaultive and agitative from an audiovisual standpoint.

The benefits of relaxation, as with nutrition and exercise, are felt on a cumulative basis. The more you practice it, the more relaxed you become. Relaxation that is refreshing, rejuvenating, and restorative requires differing amounts of quiet time from person to person. Some people may need only ten to twenty minutes to relax; others may need an hour or longer. No matter how hectic your schedule is, you can always find time to relax as long as you are willing to simplify your life by prioritizing your activities.

Use the Breath

Periodic quiet time can involve the intentional use of the breath. *Learning to use the breath is an important component of many alternative practices* and affects overall balance and harmony. The word for breath is synonymous with spirit in many cultures, and attention to the breath is a key to deepening awareness. There are many physical and mental benefits to using the breath properly and developing maximum breath capacity.

It is estimated that nine out of ten people do not breathe fully. Although our lungs have a capacity of about two gallons of air per breath, the average person takes in only a couple of pints of air at one time. An inability to breathe properly is a reflection of the stress in our lives and the mistaken assumption that beauty lies in having a flat stomach.

All cells in the body need oxygen in order to sustain life. Shallow breathing from the chest inhibits the flow of oxygen to cells in the body. Deep, slow, regular breathing from the abdomen encourages the circulation of oxygen. The former feels quite different from the latter. Notice how constricted the breath is from the chest. We are particularly inclined to breathe this way in moments of stress. Once you recognize this, you can release the breath back to the abdomen and feel instantly better.

Here are four simple ways to use the breath:

Breathing Technique #1: Sit comfortably, lightly close your eyes, and follow the breath by repeating "I am breathing in; I am breathing out." This is a basic meditation technique.

Breathing Technique #2: Sit comfortably, and lightly close your eyes. Take a full breath through the nose, hold the breath for four to eight counts, and exhale through the mouth twice as slowly as you inhaled. Pause for one moment at the end of the exhale, and repeat this process. If you are only able to hold the breath for a couple of moments at the end of the inhale, you will still benefit from the use of this technique.

Breathing Technique #3: Termed three-part breathing, sit comfortably and lightly close your eyes. First, breathe into your belly, then your lower chest, and lastly, into your upper chest. Pause for one moment at the end of the inhale. Exhale in reverse order, pause at the end of the exhale, and begin again.

Breathing Technique #4: Termed alternate nostril breathing, begin by sitting comfortably. Place your middle and index fingers between your eyebrows or curl them into your palm so that your thumb is over one nostril and your ring and little finger are over your other nostril. Lightly close your eyes. Take a breath, and close your right nostril. Exhale and inhale through your left nostril. Close your left nostril, and exhale and inhale through your right nostril. Continue alternate nostril breathing, and try to make your exhalation twice as long as the inhalation.

There are many breathwork techniques in alternative medicine that help facilitate physical, emotional, and spiritual health. Breathing techniques such as those described above are instant stress reducers and will help you to relax and fall asleep.

Breathwork is an important intervention and lifestyle change that is frequently ignored by practitioners and consumers alike. Meditation is a form of breathwork, which is described in *Step Four,* and breathwork is an integral part of inward disciplines, which are discussed in *Step Six.*

Improve Sleep

With 75% of Americans reporting sleep problems on a regular basis and only 50% reporting that they get the sleep that they need, insomnia is a pervasive disorder. It is one of the first signs of a health imbalance along with eating irregularities such as loss of appetite. It is estimated that 95% of Americans suffer from a sleep disorder such as stress-related insomnia at some time in their lives. Research shows that sleep deprivation increases the production of a dangerous stress hormone, harms brain cells, depletes the immune system, and may accelerate the aging process.

Consuming alcohol or excessive amounts of protein, sugar, and caffeine, along with strenuous physical exercise before bedtime, can inhibit the ability to fall asleep. It is also wise to avoid activities other than sleeping or having sex in your bed. Watching television or reading in bed sends a message to your brain that this location is for more stimulating activity and can adversely affect your ability to sleep. Deep breathing exercises like those described in the previous section will help you to sleep. Consuming complex carbohydrates also relaxes you for sleep. Go to bed without setting the alarm clock whenever possible. Sleeping outside in nature is the equivalent of taking a huge sedative minus the harmful side-effects.

To find out exactly how much sleep your body needs, go to bed at the same time for several nights in a row and allow yourself to wake up naturally. You will begin to awaken at the same time every morning. This is the amount of rest you need every night.

If irregular sleep is a chronic problem, you may need to rebuild confidence in your ability to sleep. More serious causes of sleep disturbance, such as an emotional disorder or medication use, require a consultation with an appropriate health care specialist.

ENVIRONMENT
"Clean Up!"

Our incessant pursuit of convenience and our embrace of competition over cooperation has resulted in an over-reliance on technology, which has caused us to pay an inevitable price for its prominence in our lives. In many instances, our use of technology supercedes common sense and good judgment.

Instead of blindly focusing on what technology can do *for us*, we should begin to recognize what technology is doing *to us*. Remember asbestos, once described as the "magic mineral," fluorocarbons, sodium saccharine, lead poisoning, and red dye #2?

Our earth is contaminated with pesticides, our oceans with refuse, our rivers with chemical waste, our atmosphere with hydrocarbons, and our food with chemical preservatives. In the spirit of capitalism and the drive to create more efficient and profitable products, did anyone ever look past the next quarterly report and ask, "Is this really good for us?" Safety is frequently sacrificed for the immediate gratification of the sale.

There are an estimated 80 million cases of foodborne illness every year, resulting in more than 300,000 hospitalizations and 5,000 deaths, and 60% of the population has developed allergies from chemical pollutants in the air, water, and food. There are concerns that excessive cell phone use and the sugar substitute Nutrasweet™ cause brain damage.

Around 10 million Americans suffer from hearing loss as a result of environmental noise, and 138 million people are regularly exposed to noise levels labeled excessive by the Environmental Protection Agency (EPA). One recent study suggests that continuous environmental noise affects speech and language development in infants. A new science termed bioacoustics has even emerged to study the negative consequences of man-made noise.

Technology is increasingly linked to serious illness, infertility, and emotional disturbance. There are an estimated 65,000 chemicals in the environment, so it is no wonder that environmental illness (EI) and multiple chemical sensitivity (MCS) have become major health concerns today. Common symptoms of environmental illness include skin disorders, fatigue, depression, and recurrent headaches. Clinical ecology, also known as environmental medicine, is the growing health care practice used to treat these illnesses and to address health concerns as they relate to home, work, and school.

Technology has become not only a hazard to our physical health but also to a rarely considered aspect of our health—our privacy. The Internet is used to track where you go, what you do, and what you buy without your knowledge or consent. Personal information is shared, and identities have been stolen.

We use machines to answer telephones, process accounts, purchase merchandise, provide information, and communicate with others. Technology has limited personal contact between human beings to the unimaginable degree that we now carry on relationships with people exclusively by machine, even when they reside nearby.

Technology has provided us with many conveniences to enhance and improve our lives, yet each innovation seems to move us a little further away from an intimate connection with ourselves and nature. Although it has enhanced commercial growth, technology has become an obstacle to personal growth. No one advocates a return to the horse and buggy or the old-fashioned icebox, but perhaps we need to begin to set limits on the extent to which technology rules our lives. Believe me, the bugs are a lot healthier for us than the bug sprays are.

In her provocatively titled book *A Cure for All Disease*, Dr. Hulda Clarke theorizes that environmental toxicity is largely responsible for most disease and is caused by two main sources—parasites in the body and pollution in the environment. New evidence suggests that parasites, previously ignored by scientists as a major factor in health, are as important as predators at the top of the food chain in all ecosystems.

Dr. Clarke believes that parasites can be eliminated and pollution can be avoided. There are many theories about the effects of environmental toxicity as public awareness of this issue continues to grow. Dr. Clarke's conclusions are disturbing not only for their extremeness but also for their plausibility.

Radical environmental lifestyle change is impractical in a modern society as dependent on technology as we are, but there are still many things you can do on your own to clean up your environment. *12 Easy Steps to Clean Up Your Environment* are:

- Reduce processed and chemically treated food from your diet.
- Prepare and store food safely.
- Drink only pure water (this usually means bottled).
- Wash your hands after handling pets and before handling food.
- Replace chemical cleaning products with nontoxic versions.
- Opt for washable floors over wall-to-wall carpet.
- Remove shoes when entering your home.
- Limit close bodily contact with electrical current (microwaves, electric blankets, heating pads, alarm clocks, etc.).
- Use an air purifier (HEPA filter, UPLA filter, or water-based system).
- Limit contact with petrochemical toxins in and around moving vehicles.
- Use cell phones sparingly.
- Reduce your exposure to noise.

Contact the American Academy of Environmental Medicine at (316) 684–5500.

2 STEP TWO
Balance Your Space
"External Energy Work"

SUMMARY & FURTHER READING

The Tao of Physics, Fritjof Capra

Consult an external energetic specialist about environmental balance. Examples are:

1. **Feng Shui**

   Interior Design with Feng Shui, Sarah Rossbach

2. **Vastu Shastra**

   Vastu Living, Kathleen Cox

"Man, you really need to *feng shui* your space!"

People are becoming more and more interested in elements outside their immediate awareness. One of these elements is the effect of energy fields on various aspects of our lives, including our health. Subtle energy refers to the vibratory fields in all living matter and is at the core of the bodymind connection. The scientific explanation of these energy fields is based on quantum physics, although many experts agree that they are difficult to measure using conventional instrumentation.

Subtle energy is known by many names: Indians call it *prana*, Tibetans call it *lung*, Hebrews call it *ruach*, and Chinese call it *qi*. It is also known as etheric energy, *fohat*, *orgone*, odic force, and *mana* among many other names. Many cultures regard it as the life force that is present in all living matter. If all animate and inanimate matter is energy in constant motion—intertwined, interacting, interconnected, and interdependent—and energy fields are believed to activate biochemical processes, the balance of subtle energy is integral to a truly holistic approach to health.

In conventional or alternative medical practice, almost no attention is given to the balance of subtle energy in the physical space as it affects health and well-being. Although alternative medicine is based on the balance and harmony of all energetic fields, it focuses almost exclusively on the flow of energy throughout the physical body and on changes in energy related to expansions of consciousness. Alternative practitioners who ignore this important aspect of health may not be aware of its existence or its import on a person's well-being, but it should be a part of every health care program. What you cannot see on the outside can definitely affect you on the inside.

The balance of energy in the physical space involves complicated spiritual practices and the use of techniques that are performed by highly skilled practitioners. There are also many things you can do on your own to balance the energy in your space. It is the first treatment suggested in the six-step plan after lifestyle factors because *if you are not in balance and harmony with your physical space, no alternative treatment or technique will be effective until balance and harmony are restored.*

Although psychic energy practices abound, there are two established practices that specifically address the balance of energy in the physical environment: the Chinese practice of *feng shui* and the Indian practice of *vastu shastra.*

FENG SHUI

A few years ago, the average person had never heard of the ancient Chinese practice of *feng shui* (pronounced fung-shway). Today, this practice is commonly featured on television and radio, in magazines and newspapers, and on the Internet. Many prominent national and international companies use *feng shui* to balance the flow of energy in their buildings, creating an atmosphere beneficial to the success of their businesses. People now use *feng shui* to design new homes and balance the flow of energy in older ones.

Feng shui, also known as geomancy, literally means wind-water. It involves divining the currents of wind and water, which reflect the movement of *qi* in the environment, and placing people in a favorable relationship to these forces. In Chinese philosophy, *qi* (pronounced chēē and also spelled chi) represents the life force. The practice of *feng shui* arose from an ancient Chinese tradition about the effects of nature and the environment on human fortune and well-being.

Feng shui addresses the rhythms of the universe according to the universal laws of nature and our interconnectedness and interdependence with those forces. When a physical space is aligned with the forces of nature or the natural flow of energy, people who occupy that space will benefit. When a physical space is disaligned with the forces of nature or the natural flow of energy, they will suffer. External space influences internal space and vice versa.

Feng shui considers the shape of the land, the cycles of weather, the flow of rivers and wind, and the patterns of sun and shade. The flow of *qi* in the natural landscape is affected by the shape and orientation of hills, mountains, and rivers. In cities, buildings are regarded as mountains and roads are viewed as rivers. *Qi* must be allowed to flow freely, slow down, meander, revolve, and accumulate. It must not be allowed to become stale, stagnate, or move too fast, causing it to disperse and scatter.

An imbalance or a misalignment with the natural flow of *qi* in a physical space creates energetic resistance, and problems can occur when this happens. When obstacles to the flow of energy are removed from a space, balance and harmony are restored to it and to the individual who occupies the space. In Chinese philosophy, there is both good and bad *qi* because energy can be positive or negative. The natural flow of energy promotes the influence of positive forces, but impediments to the natural flow promote the influence of negative forces.

There are five basic elements in the environment—fire, wood, earth, metal, and water. There are also *yin* and *yang*, the two primary forces of nature that, when combined together, create harmony. In Chinese medicine, these same forces exist within us. *Yin* is dark and passive, and *yang* is light and active. The five elements, yin, and yang are divided into different kinds of *qi* energy. The *feng shui* practitioner must determine the manner in which these elements and forces affect each other in order to align objects and activities in the environment with the movement of *qi*.

The practice of *feng shui* is used to assist in decisions on the design and placement of buildings, furnishings, business projects, and even burial sites. Furnishings are defined as any interior decor, including furniture, plants, lights, and mirrors. *Feng shui* uses light, sound, living things, heavy or electrical objects, flutes, and colors to enhance the flow of *qi* in the physical environment.

A doorway or chair is positioned in such a way that the flow of energy is enhanced in a positive manner. Windows conduct *qi* and should open completely. Lighting corrects imbalances and can activate or circulate *qi*. Mirrors provide visual expansion. Small spaces need light while large spaces can employ either dark or light. Sharp architectural angles threaten inhabitants, and a plant may be strategically placed to correct this imbalance. Driveways and roads are also important conductors of *qi*.

The practice of *feng shui* sometimes involves the balance of personal *qi*. A person can have positive or negative *qi*, like a physical space. People are susceptible to negative energetic influences such as beliefs, emotions, other people, or phenomena for a variety of reasons. The removal of bad personal *qi* requires exceptional skill. Only highly experienced *feng shui* practitioners (and *qigong* masters) perform this type of work.

Feng shui is based on the same principles as the Chinese practices of acupuncture and *qigong*. *Feng shui* addresses the flow of *qi* in the physical environment. Acupuncture and *qigong* address the flow of *qi* in and around the physical body. Same energy field; different methods. (See *Steps Three and Five*.)

It is possible to incorporate many of the basic principles of *feng shui* into your environment on your own. More complicated problems may require the assistance of a qualified *feng shui* practitioner. Practitioners of *feng shui* receive many years of training to become competent in the practice. They should possess extensive knowledge of its principles as well as intuitive skill. *Feng shui* masters possess a lifetime of experience and advanced intuitive skill. If you want to consult a qualified *feng shui* specialist, find one who has received the proper training and experience.

Acupuncturists, doctors of oriental medicine, and *qigong* practitioners may be able to refer you to a qualified *feng shui* practitioner. There are *feng shui* practitioners who will also travel to other cities and states to perform this work. Master Thomas Lin-Yun of the Black Sect Tantric Buddhist form of the practice is credited by many with popularizing *feng shui* in the West. For *feng shui* practitioners trained by Professor Lin, contact the Yun Lin Temple, 2959 Russell Street, Berkeley, California 94705, (510) 841–2347. *Feng shui* practitioners can also be found by contacting the Feng Shui Directory of Consultants at (800) 443–5894.

VASTU SHASTRA

Vastu shastra is the ancient Indian science of interior design and architecture as it relates to buildings and the environment. It is basically a Hindu form of *feng shui*. *Vastu* is based on the spiritual philosophy of the Vedas, a more than five-thousand-year-old collection of writings that describes the universal laws of nature as they apply to all life. *Vastu* was originally used to create Hindu temples according to the principles and guidelines of the Vedas. The ancient medical sciences of ayurveda, yoga, and meditation also spring from these same teachings. Ayurveda applies to the health of people, and *vastu* applies to the health of buildings or structures, similar to the relationship between acupuncture and *feng shui*.

Like *feng shui*, *vastu shastra* contains equal amounts of scientific principle and spiritual philosophy. It addresses the organization of space as it relates to the five primary elements of nature (earth, water, space, air, and fire), sun, moon, and all other elements in the universe. The honored five elements are also related to specific deities and the directions of north, south, east, and west. In *vastu*, every element in nature is irrevocably interconnected with and interdependent upon each another according to the universal law of inseparability. This is also true of the relationship between people and the environment.

The goal of *vastu* is to create harmony and balance in any physical space occupied by people in order to maximize their well-being. Physical space is arranged to reflect their connection to the flow of nature and rhythm within it. The health of a space has great impact on the health of a person. Energetic vibrations that emanate from the universe are both positive and negative, so environment and self affect each other in both positive and negative ways.

A harmonious outer space creates a harmonious inner space. If the environment surrounding a person is in perfect alignment and order, harmony is created within his body, mind, and soul. An environment organized according to the principles of *vastu* encourages the flow of nature and positive energetic vibrations within the space, which, in turn, encourages it within the person who occupies the space.

On the other hand, imbalance and disharmony in the environment result in imbalance and disharmony in the person. In other words, problems in the space create problems in the person. A disorganized environment that is misaligned with the positive forces of nature impedes the positive flow of nature within the person who occupies the space. *Vastu* attempts to enhance the positive and remove the negative vibrations from the environment. Physical spaces that are organized and aligned according to the principles of *vastu* can block or impede the flow of negative energetic forces and, therefore, minimize or eliminate their impact. *Vastu* is concerned with the structure of a building and the placement of furnishings contained within it. Emptiness in the center of a room is connected with the collection of spiritual energy, which can then be dispersed positively in every direction. Since facing east is associated with enlightenment, the head of a bed is placed in that direction to allow a person to absorb spiritual light during the night. Every environment is given an area of tranquility where a person can retreat from the stresses of the physical world. A physical space is always organized with consideration for the individual needs and preferences of the person who occupies it.

People who have organized and aligned their physical space according to the principles and philosophies of *feng shui* and *vastu* have claimed many benefits, including inner peace, improved concentration and decision-making, decreased stress and tension, improved health, and financial success. Organizing your physical space to enhance and promote your health and well-being also makes sense when you really think about it.

Like *feng shui*, you can learn about *vastu* and utilize many of the basic principles of the practice on your own. More complicated issues may require the services of a qualified *vastu* practitioner. It is also vital to find a *vastu* practitioner who is properly trained and experienced. Finding qualified practitioners of *vastu* may be more difficult than finding practitioners of *feng shui* because it is not as common in the West.

Ayurvedic practitioners may be able to refer you to a qualified practitioner of *vastu*. Centers of traditional ayurveda include the Ayurvedic Institute at (505) 291–9698, American Association of Ayurvedic Sciences (Medical Clinic) at (425) 453–8022, and Ayurveda Holistic Center and School of Ayurvedic Science at

(800) 452–1798. Centers of Maharishi Ayurveda are located in Lancaster, Massachusetts at (877) 890–8600, Fairfield, Iowa at (800) 248–9050, Dallas, Texas at (888) 259–9915, Albuquerque, New Mexico at (800) 811–0550, and Bethesda, Maryland at (301) 770–5690. The Chopra Center for Well Being, another center of Maharishi Ayurveda, can be reached at (888) 424–6772.

Other Specialists

There are many psychic energy practices. Some are merely extensions of a spiritual practice or religion; others involve individuals who claim to possess special intuitive skill. Psychic practices usually focus on the person rather than the environment. More esoteric practices that address the paranormal or psi involve removing negative energy from an environment rather than organizing your environment to promote the positive flow of energy.

Energy healing can be performed by a rabbi, priest, monk, yogi, lama, shaman or medicine man, voodoo priest or priestess, dowser, psychic, intuitive, prayer healer, or other spiritual master. There are also psychotherapists who claim to possess psychic healing ability.

Whatever the practice, qualified practitioners of energy work are extremely difficult to find. It not only takes years of training and experience but also an innate ability to effectively perceive and resolve energetic problems. But *being able to perceive an energetic problem is very different from being able to resolve an energetic problem.* There are far more practitioners who can do the former rather than the latter. As a responsible consumer, you must be able to distinguish one from the other. Resolving energetic impediments in the environment can also be hazardous work, and practitioners must take precautions to protect themselves when performing it.

There is enormous opportunity for fraud and misrepresentation in energy healing practices. Although skilled people do exist, there are those who are simply out to take your money. Remember that it is possible to believe in the power of energy work but still be skeptical of people who claim to be experts at performing it. It is prudent to exercise the same caution, if not more, in choosing an energy specialist that you would for any alternative practitioner. Remember that the use of an energetic healing practice is not a substitute for resolving other physical or emotional impediments to health.

General information on subtle energy is provided by the International Society for the Study of Subtle Energies and Energy Medicine at (303) 425–4625.

STEP THREE
Balance Your Energy
"Internal Energy Work"

SUMMARY & FURTHER READING

Choose a comprehensive medicine system to incorporate into your healing program. Examples are:

1. **Chinese Medicine**

   Between Heaven and Earth, A Guide to Chinese Medicine, Harriet Beinfield, L.Ac. and Efrem Korngold, L.Ac.

2. **Homeopathy**

   The Consumer Guide to Homeopathy, Dana Ullman, M.P.H.

3. **Ayurveda**

   Ayurveda: The Science of Self Healing, Vasant Lad M.D. (traditional ayurveda)

   Perfect Health, Deepak Chopra, M.D. (Maharishi Ayurveda)

4. **Naturopathy**

   Encyclopedia of Natural Medicine, Michael Murray, N.D. and Joseph Pizzorno, N.D.

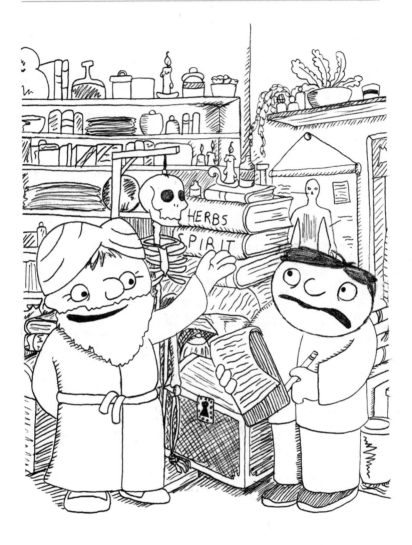

"The practice is thousands of years old!"

"I will be, too, by the time I learn it!"

The best way to achieve personal balance and harmony is to use a comprehensive alternative medicine system. These systems are designed to balance personal subtle energy through bodily intervention as opposed to the spatial intervention described in the previous step. They typically utilize a variety of modalities, methods, and techniques such as herbs, nutrition, exercise, bodywork, sensory therapies, and meditation in order to bring the body back into a state of balance and harmony.

Comprehensive systems employ a holistic approach and simultaneously consider a person's physical, psychological, and spiritual well-being. Practitioners of these systems who are properly trained will provide you with encouragement and guidance for adopting healthy lifestyle habits. They know that even the most potent treatment or natural medicine will have only limited impact if these issues are ignored.

Alternative medicine systems are based on our connection with nature, and the interventions they employ vary with both the seasons and personal change. You can regard one of these systems as your main alternative health care practice to which all other alternative treatment is a complement.

CHINESE MEDICINE

Chinese medicine has existed for more than five thousand years and is based on the principles of balancing the energetic forces of nature that are within us: heat-cold, yin-yang, and blood-qi. It can involve the use of acupuncture, herbs, diet, massage, exercise, energy work, and spiritual meditation. In Chinese medicine, prevention is equal in importance to recovery from illness. Instead of a relationship that consists of an authoritative doctor and a submissive patient, the

Chinese medicine practitioner is a partner, teacher, and participant in the entire health care process.

Health is determined by the balanced flow of *qi* in the body. In Chinese acupuncture, *qi* circulates along twelve major energy pathways known as meridians, which are connected to specific internal organs. Organs are arranged into systems, in which each organ nourishes the functioning of the other organs and systems, and are connected to one of the five elements in nature—fire, water, earth, metal, or wood.

When you are well, the energy flows freely along meridians, but when you are ill, the flow of energy along meridians is interrupted or blocked. As mentioned previously, Chinese acupuncture is the equivalent of *feng shui* for the body.

Acupuncture is the practice of inserting special, disposable needles into more than one thousand points on the body to stimulate and balance the flow of *qi* along energy meridians. The insertion of acupuncture needles feels like a small pinprick; it is painless and barely noticeable after a few sessions.

Needles may be removed immediately or left in the body for a longer period of time. The acupuncture treatment that you receive is determined by evaluating the twelve radial pulses on the wrist, skin coloring, coating on the tongue, tone of voice, nails, and particular symptomology. The initial acupuncture evaluation can take up to two hours.

Other treatments that can be performed by an acupuncturist include burning an herb called Moxa to draw *qi* to a particular acupuncture point, the use of a cup to create suction on the skin, and electrostimulation on acupuncture points. Sometimes, acupressure or Chinese massage is also incorporated into the acupuncture treatment. Although drinking alcoholic beverages is discouraged on the day of any alternative medicine treatment, this is especially true in the use of acupuncture.

Treatment with herbs, an integral part of Chinese medicine, is utilized in every traditional Chinese hospital. Herbal formulas are typically composed of anywhere from two to twenty different herbs derived from natural vegetable, animal, and mineral sources. Although the traditional method is to boil raw herbs in water to make a tea, modern Chinese herbal remedies called patent medicines are available in the form of pills, tinctures, powders, and syrups.

Be sure that the herbs you use are good quality and do not contain synthetic ingredients such as acetaminophen or dangerous chemicals such as arsenic. Chinese herbs can ameliorate the adverse effects of conventional drugs, including chemotherapeutic agents, and can be used in conjunction with conventional medicine.

Acupuncture and herbal medicine are the two most common methods of Chinese medicine available in the West. They are not always found together in the same practice because both require extensive training and experience. Chinese medicine is used for a wide variety of illnesses such as chronic pain, allergies, infertility, addiction, digestive problems, and to strengthen immunity for AIDS-related illnesses. In China, acupuncture is frequently used in place of anesthesia in medical surgery, although this practice is less common in the West.

There are many forms of acupuncture practiced today. They are all based on the same basic tenets but have slightly different approaches to treatment and emphasize the use of some techniques over others. The primary forms of acupuncture available in this country are traditional Chinese acupuncture, classical or Five Element acupuncture, which originated in England, and Japanese acupuncture. There are also significant differences in the same acupuncture practice from provider to provider because everyone has his own particular style.

Contact the American Association of Oriental Medicine at (888) 500–7999, National Certification Commission for Acupuncture and Oriental Medicine at (703) 548–9004, and American Academy of Medical Acupuncture at (323) 937–5514.

HOMEOPATHY

Homeopathy was created two hundred years ago in the late eighteenth century by a German physician named Samuel Hahnemann. Dr. Hahnemann postured three important principles in homeopathic treatment: the Law of Similars, which states that a substance in large doses produces symptoms of disease but in smaller doses will cure disease; the Law of Infinitesimal Dose, which states that the more a substance is diluted, the more potent it becomes; and the Law of Specificity, which states that illness is specific to the individual. In other words, a symptom may be the same for many people, but the way a person experiences it is totally unique to him.

Since illness is specific to the individual, homeopathic doctors take a long history during the initial appointment, which can last up to two and one-half hours. This history targets the symptoms and personal characteristics of a person, both physical and psychological. Homeopathy is unlike other comprehensive systems in that it does not employ a variety of methods and techniques. It primarily involves the prescription and application of homeopathic remedies, which correspond to particular symptoms, general physical symptoms, and psychological traits.

Homeopathic remedies are made of natural plant extracts and are formulated into sucrose pills that are then dissolved under the tongue, in the mouth, or diluted in water. Many remedies are available in tinctures for internal use as well as ointments and creams for external use. Homeopathic remedies are taken in a single dose in the doctor's office or in frequent, smaller doses at home and are manufactured in strengths appropriate for both acute and chronic conditions.

In classical homeopathy, a single remedy is utilized at one time. In other homeopathic treatment, combination remedies, in which several plant extracts are formulated together, are administered. Homeopaths use different remedies for different stages of healing because symptoms vary from stage to stage.

After a homeopathic remedy is taken, a healing crisis sometimes occurs in which a person's symptoms worsen before improving. In homeopathic practice, more recent symptoms are eliminated before older, underlying symptoms can be resolved, which is known as Hering's Law of Cure. Once the deepest underlying issue is successfully resolved, an internal energetic order is reestablished, resulting in a lasting cure.

Homeopathic remedies are known to be very effective in the resolution of conditions such as colds and flu before they become debilitating. As listed in Chapter 4, Oscillococcinum® is a popular combination remedy for the treatment of flu. Homeopathic remedies can also be used to prepare for medical surgery. Inflammatory and infectious conditions, migraines, allergies, digestive, skin, and psychological problems can be alleviated or resolved with homeopathic treatment.

Coffee, camphor (found in many lip balms), and dental work are the major antidotes for homeopathic remedies, rendering them ineffective. Treatment with homeopathic medicine requires a fair amount of vigilance and care to avoid these antidotal substances.

Due to the number of variables involved in choosing the right remedy, homeopathic treatment usually necessitates lengthy trial and error, more so than any other alternative practice. Once you take a homeopathic remedy, you may have to wait several weeks or even months to determine if it is the right one for you. If not, this process must be repeated with a new remedy until the right one is found.

Most homeopaths now use computer software specially designed for homeopathic assessment. This streamlines the diagnostic process, helping to zero in on the right remedy in a shorter period of time. Even so, homeopathy requires patience from all parties concerned. Despite these frustrations, when the right homeopathic remedy is chosen, the healing process is greatly simplified and the results can be astonishing.

Many homeopathic doctors are also medical doctors. Although experience is an important criterion in the choice of any alternative practitioner, the trial and error aspect of homeopathy makes choosing an experienced practitioner especially important. Experienced homeopaths typically charge higher fees than less experienced practitioners, but they can also save you money in the long run if they find the right remedy in less time.

Contact the National Center for Homeopathy at (703) 548-7790.

AYURVEDA

Ayurveda (pronounced ī-er-vayda) originated in India more than five thousand years ago. Many people believe that Eastern medical systems such as Chinese and Tibetan medicine are actually derived from ayurvedic practice. Ayurveda is a Sanskrit word, which means the science of life. As with Chinese medicine, prevention is as important as recovery from illness in ayurveda, and the client assumes an active role in a dynamic and equal partnership with the ayurvedic practitioner.

Ayurvedic treatment involves three basic processes— cleansing and detoxifying (*shodan*), mystical balancing and pacifying (*shaman*), and restorative tonification and rejuvenation (*rasayana*). In a comprehensive initial interview, the patient is diagnosed into one of three metabolic body types or *doshas*—*vata, pitta,* or *kapha*. Although one dosha predominates in an individual, ayurveda holds that all three are present in varying degrees throughout the body. Illness in ayurveda is defined as an imbalance among the three doshas.

Diagnosis of body type and dosha imbalance are based on the twelve radial pulses, tongue, eyes, and nails, similar to acupuncture. Ayurvedic physicians also use a urine examination to determine dosha imbalance. Each body type thrives on a specific nutritional program, exercise, lifestyle, and environment. On the basis of body type, a treatment approach is recommended using a variety of natural therapies, including nutrition, herbs, aromatherapy, music and sound therapy, exercise, yoga, meditation, and massage.

Similar to Chinese medicine and homeopathy, ayurveda addresses a wide variety of conditions. Ayurvedic practice utilizes more treatment methods and techniques at one time than other comprehensive systems, requiring more effort on your part in terms of both time and expense. On the other hand, all ayurvedic treatment methods are usually addressable with one practitioner, an advantage over other systems. Ayurvedic practitioners are generally more difficult to find because they are less common in the West than acupuncturists or homeopaths.

There are two types of ayurvedic medicine practiced in the West: traditional ayurveda, popularized by Dr. Vasant Lad of the Ayurvedic Institute in Albuquerque, New Mexico; and Maharishi Ayurveda™, created by the Hindu swami

Maharishi Mahesh Yogi of Transcendental Meditation fame and widely promoted by Dr. Deepak Chopra. Maharishi Ayurveda represents the Maharishi Mahesh Yogi's translation of the ancient Vedic texts about ayurveda. It is more common in the West and has its own line of ayurvedic products. Like most alternative practices, ayurveda was originally more mystical in its orientation than it is today. To what extent Westernized or adapted versions of ayurveda alter its overall effectiveness is unclear.

There are ayurvedic clinics in Massachusetts, New Mexico, Arizona, and California, which offer inpatient and outpatient care. For traditional ayurveda, contact the Ayurvedic Institute at (505) 291–9698, American Association of Ayurvedic Sciences (Medical Clinic) at (425) 453–8022, and Ayurveda Holistic Center and School of Ayurvedic Science at (800) 452–1798.

For Maharishi Ayurveda, contact the Maharishi Medical Centers located in Lancaster, Massachusetts at (877) 890–8600; Fairfield, Iowa at (800) 248–9050; Dallas, Texas at (888) 259–9915; Albuquerque, New Mexico at (800) 811–0550; and Bethesda, Maryland (301) 770–5690. Contact the Chopra Center for Well Being, another center of Maharishi Ayurveda, at (888) 424–6772. The College of Maharishi Ayurveda at (800) 369–6480, which offers instruction in Maharishi Ayurvedic practice, can also make referrals.

NATUROPATHY

Naturopathy originated from the European tradition of visiting health spas and natural springs in order to promote health. This trend became very popular in the United States in the mid-nineteenth century and was popularized by the

Kellogg brothers of cereal fame. Physician John Kellogg ran the Battle Creek Sanitarium in Michigan where people could "take the cure," while brother Will produced "health foods" in their factory. These early naturopaths emphasized diet and lifestyle issues and engaged in some unusual detoxification practices.

Today, naturopathy has evolved into a more reputable practice. Its principles are based on many of the Eastern medical practices such as Chinese medicine and ayurveda. Naturopaths regard illness as the body's way of dealing with a deeper underlying imbalance. If the imbalance is not removed, chronic disease results. In naturopathy, the focus is on the individual rather than the symptoms of disease. Although naturopaths usually focus on nutrition and life-style issues, they may also employ one or more therapeutic methods or techniques.

The typical visit to a naturopath requires approximately one hour and is used to assess your lifestyle and interests. Standard diagnostic tools may be administered such as a physical examination and laboratory tests. The practice of naturopathy encompasses a variety of therapies such as nutrition, exercise, herbal medicine, acupuncture, homeopathy, hydrotherapy, detoxification therapies, manipulation, counseling, and lifestyle modification. Some naturopaths use unusual methods such as bee sting therapy.

Naturopaths are generally as concerned about treating your current physical condition as they are about emphasizing long-term health maintenance. Naturopathy is best known for addressing mild, acute conditions such as colds and flu as well as chronic health conditions.

Naturopathic medicine is commonly found in the West. Although it is a comprehensive practice, the practice of naturopathy lacks consistency in training, licensing, and organization. Naturopathic practice also varies significantly from practitioner to practitioner, so you may have to search around to find one who can best serve your needs. On the other hand, naturopaths are trained to focus on lifestyle issues and healthy self-care habits, a critical factor in the promotion of good health. These preventive issues are frequently ignored by other alternative practitioners.

Contact the American Association of Naturopathic Physicians at (866) 538–2267.

Other Comprehensive Systems

Two other notable comprehensive alternative medicine systems are *Tibetan medicine* and *osteopathic medicine*. Tibetan medicine is a comprehensive system in the tradition of ayurveda. It utilizes a variety of methods and techniques, but unfortunately, there are few practitioners in the West. Contact the Chakpori Institute at (748) 641–7323 or www.tibetanmedicine.com. Osteopathic medicine is a body-specific comprehensive health care system, which is discussed in *Step Five* of the six-step plan.

Comprehensive Methods & Techniques

Many of the methods and techniques employed in comprehensive alternative medicine systems are also practices unto themselves with practitioners who specialize in their exclusive use. They include *nutritional medicine, herbal medicine, aromatherapy, music therapy, massage, yoga*, and *meditation*, some of which are discussed in other sections of this guide. *Flower essence therapy* and *sound and light therapy* are also components of comprehensive systems as well as exclusive practices. These practices merit brief mention.

The healing properties of flowers were first discovered in the early twentieth century by English physician Edward Bach. Dr. Bach identified thirty-eight different flowering plants and trees that comprise the basis for flower remedies. Flower essence therapy is the practice of ingesting the diluted essence of flowers contained in remedies in order to address emotional causes of physical and psychological problems. Progressive psychotherapists prescribe flower remedies because they address emotional issues without the side effects and complications of conventional psychotropic medicines.

Sound therapy, an integral part of ayurvedic practice, is used in many cultures to enhance the healing process. Recent research pointed to the beneficial effects of classical music on the brain, termed the "Mozart Effect," although it has yet to be replicated in other studies. Light therapy can be as simple as using full spectrum light bulbs during the winter months to alleviate the condition known as Seasonal Affective Disorder (SAD) or as complicated as using specially made light glasses to address other health problems. Sound and light are frequently combined together for therapeutic purposes.

The foundation for sound and light therapy is the belief that our senses can be utilized to effect change in our health. We know that what we eat, involving the sense of taste, has a direct impact on our health, and numerous studies have confirmed this. We have also learned that the sense of touch, through massage and other bodywork techniques, also affects our health. The healing practice of aromatherapy is based on our sense of smell. It is then logical that we might derive health benefits from using our senses of hearing and sight.

You can use comprehensive methods and techniques on your own, but for more complicated problems, you may want to consult with a qualified practitioner. Information on flower remedies can be found in *The Encyclopedia of Bach Flower Therapy* by Mechthild Scheffer. Contact the World Wide Essence Society at (978) 369–8454 and Dr. Edward Bach Center in England at 44(0)1491–834678 or www.bachcentre.com for referrals.

For sound therapy, consult the book *Sound Health* by Steven Halpern who also produces audio tapes and CDs specifically designed for healing. Consult *Mind States* by Michael Landgraf for information on the combined use of sound and light therapy. For referrals to qualified practitioners, contact the American Association for Music Therapy at (301) 589–3300 and Society for Light Treatment and Biological Rhythms at (415) 751–2758 (Fax).

STEP FOUR
Balance Your Mind
"Mind Work"

SUMMARY & FURTHER READING

Choose appropriate mindwork tools to incorporate into
your healing program. Examples are:

1. **Immune-Building Characteristics**

   *The Healer Within: The New Medicine of Mind and
   Body*, Steven Locke, M.D. and Douglas Colligan

   The Immune Power Personality, Henry Dreher

2. **Healing Attitude**

   Love, Medicine, and Miracles, Bernie Siegel, M.D.

   Teach Only Love, Gerald Jampolsky, M.D.

   Journal Writing

   At a Journal Workshop, Ira Progoff, Ph.D.

   The Family Patterns Workbook, Carolyn Foster

   Meditation

   The New Three Minute Meditator, David Harp
   and Nina Feldman (easy)

   Everywhere You Go, There You Are, Jon Kabat-
   Zinn, Ph.D. (moderate)

   How to Meditate, A Practical Guide,
   Kathleen McDonald (complex—Tibetan
   based)

3. **Hypnosis & Guided Imagery**

   Hypnotherapy, Dave Elman

   Guided Imagery for Self-Healing, Martin Rossman, M.D.

   Rituals of Healing: Using Imagery for Health and Wellness, Jeanne Achterberg, Barbara Dossey and Leslie Kolkmeier

4. **Regression Therapy**

   The Process of Healing, Alice Givens, Ph.D. (childhood/birth)

   You Have Been Here Before, Edith Fiore, Ph.D. (past life)

   Many Lives, Many Masters, Brian Weiss, M.D. (past life)

5. **Healing Connections**

   The Support Group Sourcebook, Linda L. Klein

   Self-Help Groups for Coping with Crisis, M.A. Lieberman

   Healing Words: The Power of Prayer and The Practice of Medicine, Larry Dossey, M.D.

6. **Humor**

   Anatomy of an Illness, Norman Cousins

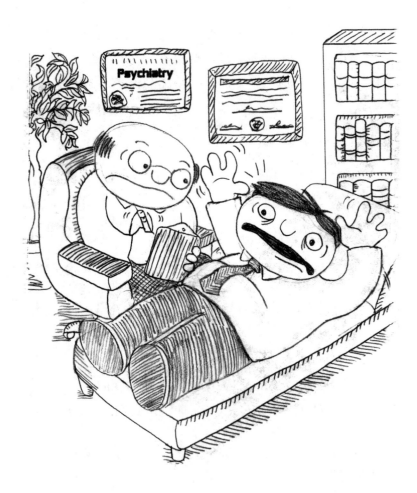

"I've tried to get over it, but I think about it morning,
noon and night; I *still* really hate eggplant!"

You are what you think, and what you think affects how you feel—this is the essence of bodymind medicine. Research shows that negative feelings, thoughts, attitudes, people, and events cause psychological stress and contribute to the development of many diseases, especially if the stress becomes chronic. Stress increases susceptibility to infection by suppressing our immunity or the body's natural ability to defend itself against foreign invaders. It is estimated that the majority of people seek medical attention for conditions that are connected to psychological stress.

Once illness occurs, negativity of any kind, a form of toxic energy, makes it very difficult to get well by obscuring knowledge of what is helpful and what is harmful for healing. Unresolved anxiety, fear, anger, and depression are often singled out as psychological states that are harmful to health. Unfortunately, the adversarial nature of our society encourages and supports many of these negative states of being. After all, criticism has been elevated into a serious and well-paid profession in politics as well as the arts.

Along the same lines, studies have shown that positive personality characteristics, attitudes, and conditions contribute to disease resistence. For example, babies who are held grow faster, smiling releases helpful hormones, and being touched lowers blood pressure. There are reports of yogis who have learned to use their mind to control bodily functions, eliminate pain, and resist infection. The capacity for joy and the ability to maintain optimism and hope are pivotal qualities for health. Faith is perhaps the most important elixir to health whether it is the ability to believe in oneself, others, the chosen treatment, a higher purpose, or a higher power.

Good health is not as simple as having positive thoughts all the time. This is an impossible feat for anyone. Having positive thoughts is beneficial, but what is more important is to learn to have a quiet mind so you have no attachment to your thoughts, whether they are positive or negative. The four cornerstones of a quiet mind are *the ability to live in the present moment, a desire to be of service to others, a nonjudgmental attitude toward life,* and *the capacity for compassion and forgiveness.* An inability to cultivate these characteristics is usually deeply rooted, requiring the greatest personal effort of all the steps in the six-step plan.

What many people discover when confronted with illness is that what used to seem important to them now seems trivial. They often report an enhanced appreciation for nature and an ability to notice it in a way they were never able to before. All sensory perceptions are heightened—colors are more vibrant and smells are more fragrant. In fact, illness allows you to become more aware of yourself and everyday life, and *developing this awareness is the key to personal growth and transformation.* Increasing awareness builds confidence and puts matters into perspective. The emotional openness that arises from increased awareness is the attitude most conducive to getting and staying well.

There is a saying that "It's easy to be a monk when you're on top of the mountain." In other words, having a loving attitude and thinking positively are easy when life is going well. When facing illness or tough times, cultivating and exhibiting these feelings are more difficult and probably the furthest thing from your mind. Changing your diet is an inconvenience, but changing your attitude is an ordeal.

Sometimes, it takes a traumatic event like illness to catapult people into examining the manner in which they regard themselves and others, as long as bitterness and anger about the predicament do not get in the way. Illness is really a great mind-opener and an extraordinary opportunity in which to expand awareness. You can definitely change your life by changing your mind.

The following psychological strategies for optimum health can be realized through a variety of interventions and practitioners—psychotherapy being only one of many options. There are also many other psychologically based techniques such as those listed in Chapter 3. Some techniques such as hypnosis are conventional; others such as regression therapy are alternative. It does not matter what label they are given if they work for you. By holistic definition, all psychological interventions impact your health and, therefore, constitute bodymind medicine. The techniques described in this step are available from psychotherapists and other health practitioners.

IMMUNE-BUILDING PERSONALITY CHARACTERISTICS

Many of the tools outlined in this step will help you to develop immune personality characteristics, which, in turn, will help you to resist and recover from disease. The science that studies this phenomenon is termed psychoneuroimmunology. Psychoneuroimmunology is specifically concerned with how the mind affects the immune system. There have been numerous studies produced in this field that demonstrate the significance of certain personality characteristics on immunity and health. These immune-building characteristics include:

- an awareness of feelings and body sensations
- the ability to confide in others
- the feeling of control over your environment
- a commitment to a personal or professional life
- the ability to regard stressful events as a challenge or gift

- assertiveness with others—refusing to take "no" for an answer

- engaging in unconditional relationships with others

- a desire to help others

- a desire for self-exploration

- the ability to tell important events from unimportant ones

- self-acceptance

- a sense of humor

- the ability to let go of anger

- feelings of optimism

According to psychoneuroimmunology, the type of person most likely to resist or recover from illness is compliant, confident, connected, commanding, communicating, and committed—the *Six C's of Health*. The person who possesses these qualities is motivated to seek health for positive reasons over negative ones like anger or revenge. A good example of turning anger and revenge into compassion is a movement called restorative or compassionate justice in which victims learn to forgive and help perpetrators of crimes that were committed against them.

If you are not born with these immune-building traits, you can acquire them by taking one step at a time. Taking small steps makes the growth process more manageable and can spark a positive chain of events to increase your power to resist and recover from illness. For example, you can gradually acquire optimism by writing down one thing every day for which you are grateful, and you can become more altruistic by regularly donating unused possessions to a thrift store.

By developing disease-resistant characteristics, the quality of your health will not only improve but so will the quality of your life.

A HEALING ATTITUDE
"Love!"

Love is the ultimate representation of a healing attitude, which you must cultivate in order to be and stay well. As the essence of spirit, love is sacred above all other things. Research supports the theory that a loving environment and a loving self-image increase the ability to be well. For many of us, disease signals the need to develop a more loving attitude toward ourselves and others. Negative feelings of fear or anger not only inhibit expressions of love but also interfere with healing.

You may be motivated by fear or anger if you:

- dwell in the past or worry about the future

- feel defensive

- find fault with yourself or others

- try to fix people or get others to fix you

- have difficulty giving or receiving

- hold a grudge

- blame people or circumstances for your problems

- need to win or be right

- avoid self-examination

- withdraw or attack others in difficult situations

When you are motivated by love, you are able to live in the present moment rather than in the past or future. You realize that giving is the same as receiving. You respect opinions that differ from your own and do not have to win, criticize, correct, attack, or humiliate another person in order to feel good about yourself. You also do not have to allow these same things to be done to you in order to feel bad about yourself.

A loving attitude allows you to feel gratitude for what you have instead of resentment about what you lack. You can forgive anything and anybody, including those who have harmed you because you are able to see another side of the situation other than your own. If you are motivated by love, you view difficult situations as opportunities for learning and growth and difficult people as teachers. You are able to surrender to the inevitability of an experience without giving up. You choose your feelings, and in choosing your feelings, you can change your perceptions.

Changes in attitude are easier said than done. When confronted with serious illness, cultivating feelings of love can feel like an insurmountable challenge. This is especially true in a social climate that values an attachment to our wounds and hanging onto negative feelings. Blame, denial, manipulation, unconstructive criticism, and aggression are all negative ways our society has learned to deal with its pain. If we truly understood how serious the consequences are to having negative thoughts, feelings, and attitudes, we might be more motivated to change them.

Many alternative practitioners will advise you to change your attitude and find a state of inner peace, but they will also provide you with little practical guidance for achieving these lofty goals. How do you surround yourself with love if you are isolated from others as many people are today, or how do you forgive someone for an irreparable injury? Many of us lack the awareness and insight necessary to achieve this kind of emotional health on our own and need help to do it.

A small step toward achieving this objective is to silently repeat affirmations when you find yourself in the center of an adversarial situation. Try repeating the phrase, "I love you," "I am peace," or "I am compassion." These affirmations are emotionally grounding and can immediately alter the dynamic of the situation.

There is much talk about awareness in our culture, but becoming or staying aware is more difficult to do than ever before in our highly externalized world. *The key to increasing awareness lies in developing an inward focus rather than an outward one.* Power exists in learning to listen to yourself.

There are many ways to cultivate a healing attitude. Three effective tools to help you change your focus, bring about psychological transformation, and achieve personal growth are talking, writing, and meditation.

Psychotherapy

Psychotherapy or counseling is the traditional method by which people in our culture heal negative attitudes and behaviors. Learning effective and loving communication skills is one of the first steps toward achieving psychological insight and a deeper level of awareness. The ability to communicate in a positive and respectful manner, which sounds deceptively easy, is often absent from our interactions with others. When you are able to communicate your thoughts and feelings in a positive way, you can alter your attitude about illness. You can also find clarity from the mere vocalization of your thoughts to another person and gain comfort from having your concerns heard.

Psychotherapy is an appropriate tool for people who require the intimacy and attentiveness of an interactive process. Its effectiveness depends on the skill of the therapist as much as your willingness to do the work. There are a multitude of psychotherapeutic techniques, traditional and nontraditional, that can help you to increase awareness. Of the tools for growth and transformation that are presented here, private psychotherapy is clearly the most costly, limiting participation to only those who can afford it.

Psychotherapy and counseling services are available from private therapists and less-costly government social service programs. The Center for Attitudinal Healing, with affiliated and unaffiliated centers around the world, provides emotional support for people dealing with illness and other disabling health conditions. They maintain regular support groups that are free and offer intensive workshops for a fee. Their program is based on many of the principles outlined above. Contact the Center for Attitudinal Healing at (415) 331–6161 for a center in your area.

Journal Writing

Therapeutic journal writing is another effective tool that allows you to gain insight into limiting beliefs and helps you to resolve conflicts that are blocking the ability to develop a positive and loving attitude. Journal writing can be as cathartic and transformational as psychotherapy, the catharsis arising from recording your thoughts and feelings on paper rather than vocalizing them.

One advantage to therapeutic journal writing is that you have the ability to reread your recorded thoughts over time, giving you a different perspective on your experiences. This affords you the opportunity to notice patterns of behavior you might not notice otherwise and gain insights from your own written word. Gratitude journals represent a popular type of therapeutic journal writing and involve keeping a daily record of all the good things in your life. Dozens of studies have found that most people feel happier and healthier after writing about traumatic experiences. A 1988 study found that it stimulated the immune system, and another one conducted in 1999 showed that it eased symptoms of asthma and arthritis. Similar writing exercises resulted in fewer trips to the doctor, better functioning in everyday tasks, and higher test scores that measure psychological well-being. Researchers believe that writing about painful experiences reduces the stress that contributes to the creation of many diseases.

When you write about your experiences, you are forced to break them down into smaller segments, making them more manageable and helping you to better understand them. Writing about your experiences can also give you a sense of control over your life. Journal writing is a valuable alternative for those who are more comfortable with the solitude of self-reflective writing than with talking therapy. For instruction in therapeutic journal writing, contact the Progoff Intensive Journal® workshops at (800) 221–5844.

Meditation

Meditation is one of the most powerful tools for inner transformation. It is an inward-focused discipline, which is found in some form in most major organized religions but is referred to by different names such as prayer, vision quest, etc. Psychotherapy and therapeutic journal writing provide a foundation for awareness and change, but meditation cultivates them on a deeper level.

There are people who will tell you that meditation is very easy. Although it is not difficult to actually perform, it is difficult to stick with it because it can take years to experience benefits other than the immediate ones of stress reduction and relaxation. Meditation requires discipline, focus, and an unwavering commitment to the process.

Simply put, meditation involves the regular training of turning the attention inward on a particular focus. The goal is to become so absorbed in the object of your attention that the superficiality of time, space, limitation, and ego fades or vanishes altogether. Meditation allows a person to observe the nature of the mind, following the ebb and flow of thoughts while being fully in the present moment. To observe the mind is to free the mind, and to be in the present moment is to be fully aware. This process leads to an understanding of the intrinsic nature of the mind. Only when the mind is calm in this way is wisdom revealed in meditation.

As the mind becomes quiet through meditation, the heart is also opened, allowing the emergence of feelings of compassion, generosity, kindness, and love even in the presence of extreme frustration and anguish. Meditation helps fine-tune the five senses, connecting people to their natural clairvoyant abilities. Some schools believe the ultimate goal of meditation is to have pure awareness without thought; others believe it is to have pure awareness simultaneous with thought. The ability of meditation to transcend ego and everyday experience distinguishes it from other personal growth and transformational tools.

Basic meditation practice involves three basic steps: (1) getting settled into position, which can be achieved by taking several deep, cleansing breaths; (2) focusing the attention or concentrating on something such as the movement of the breath or a mantra (a nonsensical word like "om"); and (3) relaxing and expanding into the meditation, the process that brings about increased awareness and insight.

Meditation can be practiced sitting, standing, walking, gazing, and lying down, and it can also include visualizations, recitations, and chanting. Within most meditation disciplines are specific exercises such as *metta*, the practice of loving-kindness, and *tonglen*, the practice of compassion. Two of the most accessible and popular meditation disciplines are: *mindfulness* or *insight meditation*, in which the attention is directed moment-by-moment to the breath and to body sensations; and *absorption meditation*, which usually involves the silent repetition of a mantra and can induce a trance-like state in which the physical world simply disappears.

Meditation can be learned from books, audio tapes, or meditation teachers, many of whom offer both group and private instruction. There are many ways to find a meditation teacher and many disciplines from which you can choose. You can also attend a meditation retreat, which lasts anywhere from one day to several weeks in length.

Contact the Insight Meditation Society at (978) 355-4378. The publication *Inquiring Mind* at P.O. Box 9999, North Berkeley Station, Berkeley, CA 94709 provides an international list of mindfulness meditation groups and workshops. Transcendental Meditation® is an absorption meditation and, like Maharishi Ayurveda, is a creation of the Indian swami Maharishi Mahesh Yogi. Contact the Transcendental Meditation center in your area by calling (888) 532-7686.

HYPNOSIS & GUIDED IMAGERY
"Imagine!"

Hypnosis

Hypnosis is usually described as an altered state of mind in which the attention is focused and awareness is heightened, not unlike meditation. The objectives are slightly different in hypnosis, which uses the power of suggestion to find the answer to a well-defined problem or to achieve a specific effect.

Whether we realize it or not, the average person experiences a hypnotic state every day—daydreaming, gazing into a flickering fire, reading a book, or driving a car on a long, straight road. The power of suggestion, which has a profound effect on the unconscious mind, can encourage deep physiological and psychological change.

Hypnosis is not what many people think it is. The hypnotic process frequently depicted in movie and television dramatizations is misleading and misrepresents how the process really works. When you are under hypnosis, you are always in control. You are completely aware of what is going on around you and can stop the hypnotic process at any time. There are also safety measures that a trained hypnotherapist can incorporate into your session to help you terminate the process if you become too uncomfortable to proceed.

The real value of hypnosis lies in its ability to provide quicker and more efficient access into the unconscious mind. The unconscious mind represents all the things that you are unaware that you already know. In psychology circles, the most common illustration of this theory is to think of your mind as an iceberg. The part of the ice above the surface of the water that you can see represents your conscious mind, and the part below the surface that you cannot see without further exploration represents your unconscious mind.

Hypnosis and variations on it are used in guided imagery, guided meditations, and breathwork. It is also the basis for regression work, which is discussed in the next section of this step. Surgical hypnosis and hypnotic anesthesia are valuable aids to relaxation and pain reduction during medical surgery.

Along with the resolution of emotional issues, hypnosis is used to treat a variety of health conditions such as anxiety, asthma, eczema, phobias, chronic pain, digestive and eliminative disorders, smoking, and weight problems.

For serious health conditions, hypnosis works best with regular use—once or more per day. Hypnotherapists, psychotherapists, guided imagery specialists, regression therapists, medical doctors, and other health care workers are trained to use hypnosis. Hypnotherapists conduct in-office sessions, create customized audiotapes for home use, and can teach you how to perform self-hypnosis. Customized audiotapes offer you the greatest ease and flexibility because you do not have to do anything but listen to the tape whenever it is convenient.

For more information on qualified hypnotherapists in your area, contact the American Society of Clinical Hypnosis at (630) 980–4740, International Medical and Dental Hypnotherapy Association (800) 257–5467, National Guild of Hypnotists at (603) 429–9438, and Milton H. Erickson Foundation at (602) 956–6196 for a list of Ericksonian-trained hypnotherapists in your area.

Guided Imagery

Guided imagery involves the use of guided meditations and visualizations in which the attention is focused on specific visual images as a way for the mind to heal the body. This technique utilizes many aspects of hypnosis and is often combined with traditional hypnosis. Like hypnosis, guided imagery can lead to a therapeutic back door, giving you quicker access to the unconscious mind than with other methods. In an indirect and a nonthreatening manner, you gain insights into limiting beliefs and attitudes and have the opportunity to adjust or alter them.

Research has shown significant health recovery benefits from the use of guided imagery. For example, burned babies healed faster with the use of guided imagery.

A popular visualization technique for healing is to close your eyes and imagine a physical form for your illness or the affected parts of your body. Surround this form or the affected parts with a comforting image like warm, golden honey or a radiant, white healing light. Many people like to visualize aggressive forms to attack and kill their illnesses. A common example of this is the use of imaginary soldiers to attack cancer cells. Adopting an aggressive, angry attitude toward illness, however, may limit the healing process instead of encouraging it.

There is a Tibetan Buddhist imagery technique termed "Feeding the Demons." This visualization involves closing your eyes and giving your illness or the affected area a physical form with as much detail as possible—eyes, nose, mouth, hair, color, and shape of the body. Then open your eyes and draw the physical form you have conjured on a piece of paper. Close your eyes again, and ask the physical form what it desires. Imagine that this desire can magically multiply into an unlimited quantity. Feed the image of your illness with its desire until it is completely satisfied. This is an example of a visualization that is based on love rather than anger toward illness.

If you are a visual person, you can use guided imagery techniques on your own. If not, you may want to consult with a guided imagery specialist who can create customized audiotapes for you to use at home. You can also create audiotapes using your own voice, a powerful therapeutic tool.

Guided imagery specialists are therapists, nurses, doctors, and other health professionals. Like hypnosis, the effectiveness of guided imagery is dependent on its regular use. Establishments that sell books, music, herbs, and natural foods usually carry visualization audiotapes and CDs. New Age publications often review them and feature the companies that make them in advertisements.

Contact the International Imagery Association at (914) 476–0781. For a referral to a specialist trained in a form of guided imagery called Interactive Guided Imagery^{SM}, contact the Academy for Guided Imagery at (800) 726–2070.

REGRESSION THERAPY
"Remember!"

Childhood & Birth Regression

Expanding awareness through the resolution of old psychological business may involve remembering events from your childhood or birth termed regression therapy. Unremembered events from the past can relate to current life problems and resulting health issues, and their rediscovery can release you from these problems. Childhood regression is universally accepted by psychotherapists as an important therapeutic tool. Birth regression is more controversial.

Many people cannot remember events from their childhood by independent recollection, especially if they are of a disturbing or traumatic nature. Few of us remember our actual birth. One tool by which people are transported into the memory of their childhood or birth is hypnosis. As discussed in the previous section, hypnosis is a technique that allows you to focus your attention with complete awareness and control. Disturbing or traumatic experiences can be remembered without any threat to your physical or emotional safety.

Amazingly minute details of childhood and birth can be recalled, and feelings, images, sounds, smells, and thoughts arise spontaneously during the regression session. In birth regression, you may recall the feelings of your mother during her pregnancy and traumatic birth or surgical experiences. In many cases, just remembering these events will release you from their power without your having to undergo wrenching analysis. When you remember events from the past, you can then process and integrate them into present experience.

Past Life Regression

Finishing old psychological business and gaining insight into current problems may involve remembering further back than you ever dreamed possible. The key to using this technique is understanding that *the answer to every question may not lie in the present lifetime.* If you have a problem that is not explainable within the context of your present lifetime, you may want to explore past life regression or the ability to remember past lifetimes.

Past life regression is more controversial for all of the obvious reasons. First, it is based on the assumption that people have lived in lifetimes other than the one in which they currently live. Second, it requires participants to suspend disbelief about their ability to move beyond this lifetime and actually remember events that occurred before birth.

People may experience moments of past life memory all the time and not realize it. *Deja vu* or the feeling that something is overly familiar can be a past life memory. Past-life experiences can be reflected in unexplainable phobias and fears or an avid interest in an unusual or uncommon vocation. An extraordinary talent or a persistent physical sensation without cause may point to a past life experience as can an ardent or unusually familiar attraction to another person.

Children have more intimate contact with spontaneous past life memory than adults because the socialization and educational process inhibits these memories as we mature.

The same therapeutic process that is used for childhood and birth regression is also used for past life regression, but the process extends beyond birth. In the same way, unresolved past life issues can release a person from destructive patterns in present day. Regression therapy also helps you to increase your natural intuitive ability.

Past life regression through the use of hypnosis with a licensed therapist is very different from past life regression that is performed by a psychic. With the former, you are the one who remembers events instead of someone else remembering them for you. There are also several breathwork techniques that can induce past life memory for the benefit of therapeutic resolution.

Two remarkable stories about past life memory recently surfaced. A young American boy recounted with great accuracy his experiences as a World War II fighter pilot, even naming all of his fallen comrades who were subsequently tracked down and found to have really existed. Since childhood, a woman in England had inexplicably drawn images of a family and village in Ireland and was haunted by their meaning. As an adult, she found the village and was reunited with elderly siblings who recognized her as their mother who had died when they were very young. Finding the adult children released her from these memories.

There are many New Age workshops on past life therapy and reports of past life experiences in the media. Although people are increasingly fascinated by the idea of past lives, regression therapy is not taken very seriously as a therapeutic technique by most psychotherapists. There was a time in the not too distant past, however, when the long-term effects of childhood problems and traumas were also not taken very seriously. To push the envelope even further, there are regression therapists who believe that people are not only capable of remembering past lives but also what happens to them in between lifetimes.

Eligibility

If the source of your current difficulties is not found in a present context, investigating unresolved issues from childhood, birth, or past lifetimes may provide answers. Regression therapy, like psychotherapy in general, is not for everyone. In fact, researchers have recently discovered that some people who revisit trauma in therapy are less well-adjusted overall than those who do not. To avoid this outcome, candidacy for participating in this work must be carefully scrutinized and assessed on an individual basis.

Most of us have the ability to be hypnotized and regressed to an earlier time. No special skill is required to participate in this easy process. The most difficult part of regression therapy is believing what you see and feel. You must be willing to accept the fact that what you are remembering is real, not fantasy or imagination. An open mind and an ability to trust the feelings, thoughts, and images that arise during the regression process are the only requirements for doing this work.

The Regression Therapist

The hypnotherapeutic skill and experience of the regression therapist are critical to the success of regression work. Therapists should only consult with clients who have thoroughly explored present lifetime issues in other therapy before initiating regression therapy. Sessions can last anywhere from one to two hours, but the regression process should not be interrupted until it is complete. Therapists should also create an atmosphere of safety for clients because of the potential for unearthing distressing events, helping them to integrate these events into present day experience.

Most, but not all, regression therapists are psychotherapists. Regression therapists are typically trained in hypnotherapy. For a referral to a regression therapist, contact the Association for Past Life Therapy at (909) 784–1570. Some hypnotherapists associated with the Erickson Institute include regression work in their practices. Contact the Milton H. Erickson Foundation at (602) 956–6196 for a list of Ericksonian-trained therapists in your area.

HEALING CONNECTIONS
"Reach Out!"

Emotional connections with others are an important part of the healing process, and research confirms it. A sense of intimacy and genuineness is at the center of all healing connections. Of course, the most positive healing connection begins with yourself. This is often the most difficult connection to make and the one most likely to be ignored or avoided. Only after you develop a positive relationship with yourself is it possible to develop healing connections with others. (See "Cultivate a Healing Attitude" in a previous section of this step.)

Developing healing connections with others is not always an easy task in a mobile, competitive society. The emphasis on technology and individual achievement makes us feel more detached than connected with others and impacts all our relationships. Detachment also affects our relationship with nature, another important healing connection. In the absence of these important relationships, people are often at loose ends and are forced to create opportunities for fellowship that are more and more contrived.

Healing connections include self-love, the support of loving family and friends, a positive relationship with a health practitioner, satisfying work, an intimate bond with nature, a close attachment to an animal, and faith in a higher power. Healing connections can also involve support groups and the power of prayer.

Support Groups

The presence of social supports has been linked with greater immunity, and support group participation has resulted in positive outcomes for both coronary heart disease and breast cancer patients. Although social support can emanate from a positive relationship with anyone, group support is beneficial in other ways. A special bond is created among individuals who are dealing with the same health problem and have similar goals for its resolution. A support group environment also allows you to know that you are not alone in this effort.

Since support group participants have similar goals, they are an important source of health information about experiences with providers, the pros and cons of treatment, self-care issues, and alternative medicine options. Barriers to healing can be both tangible and intangible. Support group participants understand this because their circumstances force them to, and the collective force of this understanding is not only comforting but also powerful in its potential to create positive change.

If you already possess a strong support system, you may not need to seek outside support. People whose support system is scattered to the four winds can stay connected to the people they care about through a free Internet-based service called CaringBridge. This service provides personalized web pages to people dealing with prolonged medical care or illness, which can then be confidentially accessed by long-distance family and friends.

If your support system is not strong, you may want to consider joining a support group. Organizations such as the Cancer Society, Arthritis Foundation, Diabetes Society, and Kidney Foundation provide information about support groups for the conditions they represent, and many of them have both local and national chapters. Information about local support groups is also available from hospitals, health agencies, social service programs, public libraries, and churches. The Center for Attitudinal Healing, referred to earlier in this step, provides free group support to people with any health issue, including chronic and life-threatening illness and the disabled. They also offer support for the bereaved and caretakers of those who are ill.

Prayer

Prayer is really just a spiritual form of group support. A recent study suggested that intercessory prayer, or prayer performed by one person to benefit another, has health benefits for people with heart disease. Religious and spiritual groups provide social supports and offer spiritual interventions to assist members and others in their quest for healing. They maintain prayer circles and telephone chains, in which members call one another to pray for your healing. Eastern religious practices like Buddhism and Hinduism offer healing rituals or ceremonies, chanting, and bell ringing—usually for a small fee or donation. Spiritual healing interventions like these are usually open to everyone, regardless of membership or spiritual affiliation.

HUMOR
"Lighten Up!"

No mention of the therapeutic benefits of humor can be made without reference to Norman Cousins, who brought attention to this often-overlooked therapeutic tool in his best-selling book *Anatomy of an Illness*. Mr. Cousins believed that he was able to recover from a connective tissue disease through the use of humor as a healing intervention. In the early 1900s, the psychiatrist Sigmund Freud wrote about the health benefits of humor. More recently, scientific research confirmed the physiological benefits of humor and its effectiveness as a stress management tool.

Humor is a very grave matter. Writer James Thurber once said, "Humor is emotional chaos remembered in tranquility." A lack of humor causes us to take ourselves and our lives too seriously, and sadly, there are many people with little or no humor in their lives. A sense of humor is a simple, inexpensive tool to use but a difficult one to acquire if you do not already possess it. A recent study suggested that humor is learned rather than innate or genetic, which suggests that it is never too late to develop a sense of humor. Since emotional benefit equals physical benefit, laughter may indeed be part of the cure for what ails us.

Norman Cousins found humor in Marx Brothers' movies. Whether you watch episodes of *The Three Stooges*, frequent comedy clubs, read comic strips, or surround yourself with people who have a well-developed sense of humor, there is nothing more therapeutic than a good laugh or being able to see the funny side of life's most challenging moments. A healing attitude, described earlier, generates a change in perception. Since perception is a choice, you can choose to perceive life with solemnity or levity. In others words, the healing process may be greatly advanced if you are simply willing to "lighten up."

Humor is used as an expression of both affection and grief. Finding humor in tragedy does not mean that you have a lack of respect for the need to grieve a loss or misfortune. When humor is appropriately applied to tragic circumstances, it is always based on love and kindness, never cruelty, and becomes cathartic and healing. Humor that is cruel is based on fear and anger and does not promote healing.

Being able to see a lighter side to personal difficulties encourages movement in a positive forward direction. Humor has the ability to put life and life-altering events into perspective, providing a positive lens through which you can view the world.

Contact the American Association for Therapeutic Humor at (314) 863-6232. The Laughter Therapy Foundation at Box 827, Monterey, California 93942 distributes special videotapes of the television program *Candid Camera* to people who are ill. The Laughter Heals Foundation at (818) 990-2019 provides services to groups, facilities, and health professionals.

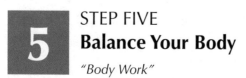

STEP FIVE
Balance Your Body
"Body Work"

SUMMARY & FURTHER READING

Choose appropriate bodywork therapies to incorporate into your healing program. Examples are:

1. **Massage Therapy**

   The Massage Book, George Downing

2. **Craniosacral Therapy**

   Your Inner Physician and You: Craniosacral Therapy Somatoemotional Release, John E. Upledger, D.O.

3. **Feldenkrais Method**

   The Potent Self: A Guide to Spontaneity, Moshe Feldenkrais and M. Kimmey

4. **Polarity**

   A Guide to Polarity Therapy: The Gentle Art of Hands-On Healing, Maruti Seidman

5. **Medical Qigong**

   The Most Profound Medicine, Roger Janke

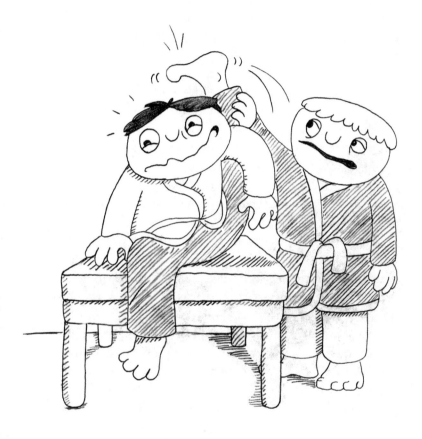

"Does it hurt when you do...*this?*"

Bodywork is a widely used and accepted health care practice in many societies. It is one of the fastest growing professions in alternative medicine. In its many forms, it can be massage, deep tissue, pressure point, movement integration, psychological, and energetic.

Bodywork that is combined with psychotherapy or emotional release is termed somatic bodywork or body psychotherapy. Somatic bodywork, which is the current trend, addresses physical and emotional restriction and limitation at one time.

There are countless bodywork therapies in the alternative medicine marketplace. They range from the conventional such as applied kinesiology to the controversial such as magnetic field therapy. Many bodywork therapies such as Trager and Reichian are incorporated into massage practices; other therapies such as the Alexander Technique, Rosen Method, and Rolfing are typically practiced on their own. Most bodyworkers employ a combination of methods and techniques in their practices.

Most bodywork involves hands-on therapy; other bodywork practices such as Medical Qigong do not involve touching the body at all. In general, bodywork reduces pain, increases overall awareness, improves biological function, promotes relaxation, and restores balance to the individual in order to encourage the healing process.

Bodywork is performed by osteopaths (DO), chiropractors (DC), physical therapists (RPT), certified bodyworkers, and massage therapists (CMT). Bodywork practitioners receive either a license to practice issued by the state in which they reside or certification in the particular bodywork therapy. Training and experience requirements for bodywork differ from method to method and vary in length from a few weeks to several years.

The services of osteopaths and chiropractors are covered by most health plans, but other practices such as massage therapy require a prescription from a medical doctor in order to be eligible for insurance benefits.

Osteopathic Medicine

Osteopathic medicine is a comprehensive system with a focus on physical medicine. It was developed as an alternative to the medical practices of the late 1900s and literally means bone suffering. Osteopaths consider themselves on a par with medical doctors. In fact, their training is very similar, and they perform many of the same functions as medical doctors. Osteopaths can be primary care physicians or general physicians, ordering diagnostic tests and prescribing drugs. They can have hospital privileges, perform surgery, and deliver babies. There are also many osteopaths who do not perform any of these functions and focus exclusively on performing hands-on bodywork.

Osteopathic medicine promotes a holistic viewpoint and an emphasis on the musculoskeletal system. The main role of an osteopath is to use the physical structures of the body to facilitate the natural tendency toward health and healing. Using their hands, they touch living tissue in order to facilitate change. Osteopathy also emphasizes self-healing and health maintenance. All osteopaths receive training in craniosacral therapy, which is discussed below. They perform soft tissue and spinal manipulation. Some osteopaths practice magnetic field therapy, which involves the use of magnets to alleviate physical pain.

Contact the American Osteopathic Association at (800) 621–1773 and American Academy of Osteopathy at (317) 879–1881 for osteopaths. Contact the Bio-Electro-Magnetics Institute (775) 827–9099 for information on magnet therapy.

MASSAGE THERAPY

The benefits of massage are numerous. Massage can reduce pain, increase circulation, reduce swelling, promote relaxation, facilitate elimination, release tension, and stimulate organs. Research found that babies who were massaged grew faster than babies who were not massaged. Massage can reduce blood pressure, boost the immune system, reduce harmful stress hormones, ease inflammation, stimulate nerves that carry signals to the brain, alter brain waves, and increase helpful brain chemicals such as serotonin.

Not only are there physiological benefits from massage, but it is also mentally relaxing, helping to quiet the mind. Massage also constitutes a type of one-way intimacy. You get the physical pleasure of being stroked in appropriate ways without obligation or reciprocation other than a simple fee for service.

There are many forms of massage therapy, and most massage therapists use a combination of methods in their practices. The two most common massage methods are *Swedish*, which employs long, deep strokes, and *Shiatsu* from China, which applies pressure along energy meridians and acupressure points to stimulate the flow of energy and relax the body.

Reflexology, performed by most massage therapists, is the stimulation of specific points on the foot that correspond to specific organs, which, in turn, are stimulated. *Deep tissue*, also known as sports massage, focuses attention on a particular area of the body, addressing all of the underlying soft tissues. Contrary to popular opinion, deep tissue massage does not always involve deep pressure. *Jin Shin Jyutsu* (pronounced jin-shin-jitsu) is a Japanese pressure point technique like Shiatsu, only the acupressure points are held longer.

Different conditions require different methods of massage. For example, Swedish massage is used for relaxation, but rehabilitation from an injury may require deep tissue methods.

The Chinese regard massage with unusual reverence. There are Chinese doctors who specialize in massage, and traditional Chinese hospitals offer massage as routine treatment. Along with Shiatsu, there are other methods of massage from China. *Tui-Na* is a bodywork practice that involves the back of the wrist, heel, and palm of the hand on tender reflex points and muscles and includes the use of acupressure, manipulation, and massage. *Chi Nei Tsang* (pronounced che-ney-sang) is an abdominal massage that improves digestion, congestion, immunity, and promotes circulation for the entire body.

Although Swedish, Chinese, and Japanese massage are the most commonly known methods, there are two established forms of traditional Thai massage used for medicinal purposes. *Naud Bo Rarn* combines stretching with pressure points along the body but with particular emphasis on the legs. *Jop Sen* is regarded as a more precise form of massage, which uses pressure points for more rapid healing. *Jop Sen* was originally used by royalty and high-ranking military personnel and is not widely practiced today.

Approximately one-half of the states license massage, and certification is available from the National Certification Board for Therapeutic Massage and Bodywork.

Conventional doctors, orthopedic surgeons, osteopaths, alternative practitioners, chiropractors, and physical therapists make referrals to qualified massage practitioners. *Massage Magazine* at (916) 757–6033 has information on workshops and massage therapy. Contact the American Massage Therapy Association at (847) 864–0123, American Oriental Bodywork Therapy Association (856) 782–1616, and International Massage Association at (540) 351–0800.

CRANIOSACRAL THERAPY

Craniosacral therapy is based on the functioning or dysfunctioning of the craniosacral rhythm, which is used to determine if there are restrictions in the craniosacral system. Cranial refers to the cranium or head, and sacral refers to the base of the spine and tailbone. The craniosacral rhythm is the increase and decrease of cerebrospinal fluid in and around the craniosacral system.

Imbalances in the craniosacral system are believed to occur at birth, with physical injury, and from other imbalances in the body. Therapeutic treatment involves gentle hands-on manipulation of the underlying meninges, which enclose the brain, spinal cord, and spinal fluid, to remove restrictions. Other forms of cranial therapy involve the manipulation of the sutures and nerve endings in the skull.

Craniosacral therapy increases the functioning of the central nervous system and has been successful in treating conditions, such as migraines, dyslexia, epilepsy, stroke, temporomandibular joint syndrome, mood disorders, and cerebral palsy. Researchers are currently investigating the scientific aspects of the craniosacral system.

Craniosacral therapy has been practiced by osteopaths for decades as cranial osteopathy but was only recently popularized by the osteopathic physician John Upledger. The Upledger Institute trains other types of practitioners, including registered physical therapists and massage therapists, in this method. This has generated controversy in the bodywork industry and has alienated Dr. Upledger from many of his osteopathic colleagues who believe that only they receive the necessary training to perform this technique. The practitioners who perform craniosacral therapy, however, believe it is an important and effective adjunct to their work.

Contact the osteopathic medicine associations listed in the section above or the Upledger Institute at (561) 622-4334 for referrals.

FELDENKRAIS METHOD

Moshe Feldenkrais, a former physicist, created the Feldenkrais Method as a result of his own sports-related injury. This method of bodywork is based on the movement, thought, and feeling patterns that are acquired over the years as a result of one's self-image. The Feldenkrais Method assumes that these positive and negative patterns become familiar to us and can cause both physical and emotional problems.

The Feldenkrais Method is taught in two basic ways: group instruction, which is termed Awareness through Movement® and involves a sequence of movements that are designed to replace old patterns of movement; and individual instruction, which is termed Functional Integration® and involves learning new patterns of movement through individualized touch. With either approach, the proper use of the breath and the observation of movement increases awareness, causing movement to improve and allowing old negative patterns to be replaced with positive ones.

The Feldenkrais Method is designed to allow people to move more easily without imposing a particular style on them. It is beneficial with athletic performance, back problems, and restrictions in movement. Although Feldenkrais has been successfully used to treat physically debilitating accidents and illnesses, this practice concerns itself more with the person than the injury or illness.

Contact the Feldenkrais Guild of North America at (800) 775-2118 for information.

POLARITY THERAPY

Polarity Therapy was developed by Randolph Stone, a chiropractor, osteopath, and naturopath. This method is based on the electromagnetic energy fields of the body in the tradition of Eastern methods such as Chinese acupuncture and addresses imbalances in the flow of subtle energy. In Polarity Therapy, the hands, one as a positive and the other as a negative, are used to release energy blockages by manipulating pressure points and joints in the body.

Massage, breathing, exercise, and nutrition are all components of Polarity Therapy and affect a person's physical, emotional, and spiritual condition. Since this bodywork method was designed to resolve general energetic imbalances, it is used to treat a variety of conditions and illnesses safely and effectively.

Contact the American Polarity Therapy Association (303) 545–2080 for referrals.

MEDICAL QIGONG

Medical Qigong (pronounced chēē-gong and also known as external *qigong*) is an advanced energetic practice, which is not widely available in the West. It is based on the Chinese practice of *qigong,* which anyone can learn as a regular inward discipline and whose benefits are discussed in the next step. When performed on people by qualified practitioners for the purpose of healing, the practice becomes known as Medical Qigong.

Medical Qigong facilitates the resolution of internal energetic imbalance from outside the body, much like an external form of acupuncture. Promoting the flow of *qi* or life force in the body, the *qigong* master uses his own energy field to repair and heal the flow of energy in another person. He does this by moving his hands on the outside of the body, usually without coming in contact with the body at all. In order to receive the maximum benefits of Medical Qigong, you must engage in the simultaneous daily practice of *qigong*.

On the surface, this powerful healing practice resembles the techniques of spiritual and psychic healers. Unlike the religious laying on of hands, however, the practitioner's hands are in constant motion in Medical Qigong.

There are also two Western techniques similar in appearance to Medical Qigong: *Therapeutic Touch*[SM], which is reportedly used by registered nurses in 80 hospitals in North America; and *Energy Healing*, which is practiced at Columbia-Presbyterian Hospital in New York City and California Pacific Medical Center in San Francisco. Both of these techniques utilize the hands to manipulate human energy fields in order to affect health, but Medical Qigong is the more established practice. A recent study found little benefit from the use of Therapeutic Touch, but keep in mind that the efficacy of any energy work is almost entirely dependant on the skill of the practitioner.

Many years of practice are required to become a *qigong* master, and only the most experienced practitioners perform *qigong* on others. Although Medical Qigong is not widely available in the West, there are several practitioners in California. As an element of Chinese Medicine, doctors of oriental medicine may practice Medical Qigong or they may be able to refer you to a qualified practitioner.

Contact the National Qigong Association (218) 365–6330, International Institute of Medical Qigong (831) 646–9399, and World Society of Medical Qi-Gong at 9 Hepingjie Beikou, Chaoyang District, Beijing 100013, People's Republic of China, phone number 86–1–4211591.

STEP SIX
Prevent Future Imbalance
"Soul Work"

SUMMARY & FURTHER READING

Care of the Soul, Thomas Moore

The Seat of the Soul, Gary Zukov

Initiate the regular practice of an inward discipline. Examples are:

1. **Meditation**

   The New Three Minute Meditator, David Harp and Nina Feldman (easy)

   Everywhere You Go, There You Are, Jon Kabat-Zinn, Ph.D. (moderate)

   How to Meditate, A Practical Guide, Kathleen McDonald (complex—Tibetan-based)

2. **Yoga**

   Yoga Journal's Yoga Basics: The Essential Beginner's Guide, Mara Carrico and *Yoga Journal*

   Yoga Mind and Body, Sivananda Yoga Center

   American Yoga Association Beginner's Manual, Alice Christensen

3. **Tai Chi**

    Ultimate Guide to Tai Chi, edited by John R. Little and Curtis F. Wong

    Tai Chi for Health, Edward Maisel

    Tai Chi for Beginners, Claire Hooton

4. **Qigong**

    The Way of Qigong: The Art and Science of Chinese Energy Healing, Kenneth S. Cohen

    Qi Gong for Beginners, Stanley D. Wilson

    Qigong for Health and Vitality, Michael Tse

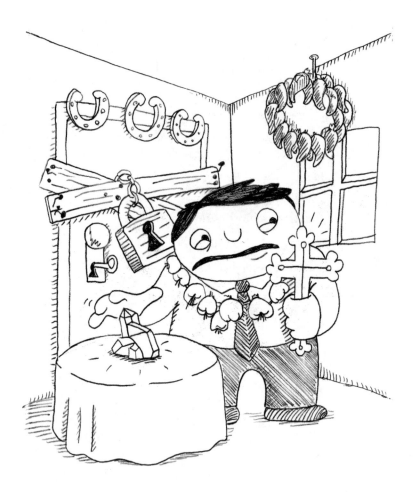

"Nothing can get to me here!"

The development of an inner life is perhaps the most important step toward healing because the most profound awareness arises from the silence of going within. Inward disciplines, which are also termed contemplative practices, advance physical, emotional, and spiritual awareness and health. The benefits of an inward discipline accrue with daily practice and with the depth of your commitment to it. Breathwork comprises the core of almost all contemplative practices.

The practice of an inward discipline is a healing intervention in and of itself and maximizes the benefits of all alternative medicine. This is the reason why it is so important to begin an inward practice as soon as possible in any serious health care program.

Although you can learn an inward practice on your own, it is more advantageous to receive instruction, at least initially, from an experienced teacher. Teachers can answer questions, correct misperceptions, and get you started on the right path. The ultimate purpose of an inward discipline, however, is to regularly practice it on your own. Relying exclusively on teachers and participation in classes transforms inward disciplines into an infrequent physical and mental exercise. Although physical or mental fitness may be an outcome of using an inward practice, this is not its primary goal.

Choose an inward discipline that appeals to you. To find a discipline that is right for you, read about it, discuss it with knowledgeable people, and attend classes that accommodate beginners and are taught by qualified instructors. Most instructors will allow you to try a class free of charge or for a modest drop-in fee or donation.

There are also many forms of each inward discipline. For example, there are six main branches of yoga practice, each representing a different focus: wisdom, meditation, physical, action, devotion, and energy awakening. The branch most commonly found in yoga classes is hatha yoga (physical), but there are also many schools of hatha yoga, which may be defined by a particular teacher or guru. These include iyengar, ashtanga, bikram, viniyoga, sinvananda, and kundalini.

Yoga is also a lifestyle, not merely a physical exercise, which is true for most inward disciplines. The complete practice of yoga involves meditation, nutrition, relaxation, breathwork, service, and cultivating a balanced state of mind.

Inward disciplines defy universal description because every person experiences them differently and because they are comprised of so many components. Teachers often advise students to avoid comparisons and extensive discussion about their practice with others. By keeping your practice private, you honor the uniqueness of your own experiences.

Most contemplative practices involve highly complex movements, however, meditation is the exception to this rule. (See *Step Four* "A Healing Attitude.") What inward disciplines do have in common is their ability to provide protection from physical, mental, and spiritual imbalance and give purpose and meaning to the experience of illness.

Engaging in an inward discipline used to be an activity of choice rather than a necessity and was only embraced by New Age types and other nonconformists. Sensible people did not have time for it, even when they became ill. This is no longer true. The practice of an inward discipline has not only become a beacon for people with anti-aging concerns but is also essential to being and staying well.

Protection & Prevention

If you are serious about being well, inward disciplines help you to achieve this goal. They provide protection from disabling influences of all kinds. They preserve the balance that is achieved through the use of interventions such as those described in the previous steps. The practices that employ movement also improve physical fitness, increasing strength, endurance, and flexibility. All inward disciplines promote relaxation.

Inward disciplines are also therapeutic in and of themselves. Studies show that meditation contributes to the reduction of chronic pain and yoga aids respiratory function. Inward practices reduce anxiety, stress, blood pressure, heart rate, and improve metabolic function, motor skills, memory, and perception.

Once you recover from an imbalance, inward disciplines help you to avert or withstand another one. When an imbalance begins to occur, the body has many ways to signal you that something is wrong. Most of us ignore these signals, if we notice them at all, until our condition becomes much worse, and we are forced to deal with it. When you develop awareness through the use of an inward discipline, you will be alert to an imbalance long before it escalates into a crisis state.

Purpose & Meaning

Inward disciplines provide purpose and meaning to life by placing your experiences into a larger context. They make life more manageable and provide a supportive environment for doing all other work. Inward disciplines aid the development of a meaningful spiritual life. They provide pathways to inner peace, reflection, clarity, spontaneity, compassion, love, and kindness—all important components of health.

Inward work nurtures the soul and cultivates presence. It encourages spiritual growth by allowing you to develop other states of consciousness. Spiritual growth leads to spiritual enlightenment and a state of bliss, often referred to as "heaven on earth." The regular practice of an inward discipline improves the quality of life in wellness and illness.

For information on yoga, contact the American Yoga Association at (941) 927–4977, Yoga Alliance at (877) 964–2255, and Yoga Research and Education Center at (707) 928–9898. For information on *tai chi*, contact the American Foundation of Traditional Chinese Medicine at (415) 776–0502. For information on *qigong*, contact the National Qigong Association at (888) 233–3655. For information on meditation contact the organizations listed in *Step Four*. There are also nationally circulated magazines that contain helpful information about these disciplines, such as *Yoga Journal* at (510) 841–9200, *Tai Chi Magazine* at (213) 665–7773, and *Qigong Magazine* at (800) 824–2433.

CHAPTER 6

USE ALTERNATIVE MEDICINE
TO SURVIVE SURGERY

M edical surgery is both psychologically intimidating and physically traumatic. There are many alternative medicine methods and bodymind techniques that can be utilized before, during, and after medical surgery to ameliorate its effects and enhance your ability to heal from it. You can adapt any alternative method or technique to the operating room and hospital environment. Methods and techniques that can be used for medical surgery include herbs and supplements, aromatherapy, guided meditations and imagery, music therapy, positive affirmations and statements, and emotional support.

To prepare for surgery, develop a positive relationship with your medical surgeon and meet your anesthesiologist. Sometimes, this is more difficult than it sounds, but unless you are in an emergency situation, you should insist on getting to know both of them. As the man in charge, your surgeon can ensure that you have the atmosphere you need in the operating room. He should know the alternative methods and techniques you intend to use to confirm that

they do not interfere with his ability to do his job successfully. The anesthesiologist is a valuable ally because he can
facilitate your use of bodymind techniques during the actual
surgical procedure.

Herbs & Supplements

There are Western and Eastern herbs that will both protect
you and help you to heal before and after surgery. As discussed previously, herbs come in many forms—dried for teas,
tinctures, extracts, tonics, pills, powders, creams, oils, ointments, and in a raw natural state. Some are more effective
when taken before rather than after surgery because they
bolster your body's natural ability to defend itself and prepare it to withstand the shock of the surgical procedure.

Unless you are knowledgeable about herbs and have
extensive experience using them for medicinal purposes,
consult with a qualified herbalist to ensure that you get the
appropriate remedy and dosage for your needs. This is especially important because with medical surgery you do not get
a second chance to get it right.

There are alternative remedies and herbs specific to
physical and emotional trauma. They include the Chinese patent medicine *Recovery*, Bach Flower remedy *Rescue
Remedy*®, and a similar flower essence combination *Five
Flower Formula*™. The homeopathic medicine *arnica*, in its
most diluted form, is effective in the treatment of physical trauma, reducing the muscle soreness that usually results
from surgery.

There are a variety of Western and Eastern herbs you
can use individually or in combinations to calm and relax
the body, support and enhance the immune system, protect
against infection, and promote healing. Sleep, which is so

essential to recovery, can be enhanced with herbs such as *valerian, hops, passion flower,* and *scullcap* in various combination formulas. Supplement formulas, such as the *Wellness Formula*® by Source Naturals and *Advanced Immune Building System*™ by Rainbow Light, are specifically designed to support the immune system.

Liquid vitamin E, calendula, echinachea, comfry, gotu kola, and the Chinese patent medicine *Yunnan Pai Yao* are all topical remedies for incision or wound healing. *Acidophilus* restores the natural flora of the digestive and intestinal tracks, which can be damaged by antibiotics given to you during and after surgery. *Ginger* reduces or eliminates nausea from postoperative drugs such as antibiotics, pain medication, and chemotherapeutic agents.

Alternative medicine remedies, herbs, and supplements can be purchased at the locations that are listed in Chapter 4. Contact the organizations listed at the end of that chapter for more information.

Aromatherapy

Aromatherapy is the practice of releasing and inhaling the aroma of essential oils, which are distilled primarily from flowers and plants. Essential oils have specific biochemical attributes that have a therapeutic effect on a range of physical and emotional conditions from infectious disorders to stress-related illnesses. Aromatherapy is widely practiced in Europe, especially in France. It is an integral part of ayurvedic practice, although there are many practitioners who specialize in the exclusive use of this technique.

There are many health benefits to using aromatherapy for medical surgery. For example, *lavender, chamomile,* and *ylang ylang* relieve mental and physical stress, helping you to relax before and after surgery. *Tea tree, rosemary, clove,* and *cinnamon* strengthen and stimulate the immune system, helping the body to resist infection.

Essentials oils are usually applied externally. They are typically applied directly onto the skin, particularly under the nose or at the temples. They can also be placed in massage oil, on a cloth, which is then applied to the body, or added to a warm bath. Although essential oils are usually inhaled, they can also be taken internally with proper supervision. An example of an essential oil taken internally is spearmint, which is commonly found in dental toothpastes and mouthwashes.

Inhalation of the aroma of essential oils is usually accomplished with the use of an aromatic diffuser, which volatizes the oils. Diffusers range from simple contraptions to more complex electrical machines that disperse the essential oil with a fan or heating element. Aromatherapy lamps also diffuse essential oils by heating them with a candle in a specially designed clay pot. Heating elements can overheat the essential oil, however, altering its chemical structure and potency.

The practice of aromatherapy is highly individualized— what is pleasing to one person may be unpleasant to another. As a general rule, you should choose essential oils whose scent is personally appealing to you because what appeals to you is probably what your body needs.

Pure essential oils, although more expensive, are preferable to ones that are diluted. Essential oils are also available in blends in which several oils are combined together in the same formula. Like any herb or herbal remedy, problems can occur with their improper use.

Essential oils can be purchased at any location where alternative remedies and herbs are sold. Contact the National Association for Holistic Aromatherapy at (888) 275–6242 or Pacific Institute of Aromatherapy at (415) 479–9121.

Guided Meditations & Imagery

As mentioned in *Step Four*, studies suggest that guided imagery has many health benefits. One study showed that the use of guided imagery (and music) made for happier patients who were discharged from the hospital sooner. Being in a relaxed and positive state of mind will help you to prepare for and recover from surgery as well as ensure a successful surgical outcome. Certain sights, suggestions, and sounds can also assist you in achieving these goals.

Guided meditations and imagery include not only meditations and visualizations but any suggestions that are positive and helpful to you. A guided meditation may take you on a relaxing visual journey through meadows, around mountains, and along streams with soothing music played in the background. Guided imagery may involve using images to increase blood flow to the affected area of the body or to strengthen T cells.

You can create your own guided meditations and imagery; purchase commercially produced audio tapes, compact discs, and books on meditations and imagery; or consult with a psychotherapist, hypnotherapist, or other health provider who specializes in these techniques and can tailor them to your own particular needs. If you have an audio player with a record feature and microphone, you can record meditations and imagery using your own voice, a powerful healing mechanism. You can also employ the services of a surgical hypnotherapist who will accompany you to surgery, placing you in a hypnotic state and making helpful suggestions to your unconscious mind when you are under anesthesia.

Guided meditation and imagery cassette tapes, compact discs, and books containing meditation and imagery scripts are available from a variety of sources. Consult your local or online bookstore, music store, and natural food store. New

Age periodicals also include resources for meditation and imagery tools. Contact the organizations listed in *Step Four* under "Hypnosis & Guided Imagery" for more information.

Music Therapy

Music therapy, which typically involves New Age or classical music, is defined as the use of music and sound to promote health and healing. Music played openly during surgery creates a pleasant atmosphere for everyone, including the surgical team.

Studies demonstrate the health benefits of music, including improvements in overall self-concept, spatial and temporal reasoning ability, and academic achievement. One study showed an increase in a family of proteins associated with blood and platelet production, lymphocyte stimulation, and cellular protection termed the "Mozart Effect." Scientists are also trying to determine if certain sounds result in the necessity for less pain medication and fewer side effects from treatment.

During surgery, music can be played openly on a boombox, portable cassette player, or compact disc player with a headset. Most surgeons routinely play music in the operating room and are usually willing to play your tapes on their stereos. If you let the surgeon play his own music, make sure it is pleasurable to you as well as conducive to getting the best outcome from surgery.

Using a portable cassette or compact disc player with a headset allows you to simultaneously block out normal operating room noise. To do this, however, you must remain in one physical position throughout the surgery or have the anesthesiologist adjust the audio player for you when you are moved. An auto reverse feature allows you to play music continuously unless your anesthesiologist is also willing to replace or rewind the tape or disc for you when it stops.

Music specifically designed for healing is available in cassette and compact disc formats from the same sources as those listed previously for guided meditation and imagery. Contact the American Association for Music Therapy at (301) 589–3300.

Positive Affirmations & Statements

Affirmations are statements that are designed to encourage a positive state of mind so that your body is supported in doing the work it needs to do to facilitate surgery and the recovery process. Your surgeon, anesthesiologist, or surgical hypnotherapist can say positive affirmations aloud to you when you are going under anesthesia and at the conclusion of surgery. You can also say affirmations to yourself before and after surgery.

Affirmations appropriate for surgery include statements such as "You are comfortable and relaxed," "Your immune system is strong," and "You will heal quickly." The most effective affirmations are the ones you create yourself. If someone else is saying them to you, ask him to personalize the statements by adding your name as in "Susie, you are comfortable and relaxed."

Please note that an absence of negativity is absolutely critical to the success of medical surgery. It is important for your surgeon to understand this and to convey it to every member of the surgical team, so they will refrain from making negative comments in the operating room. Although you can block out most sounds with the use of an audio player headset, there is no guarantee that you will be unaffected by such comments during the procedure. Most surgeons understand the need for a positive surgical environment and will accommodate your request.

In addition to positive affirmations of your own design, you can purchase cassette tapes, compact discs, and books of affirmations from the same sources as those listed previously for guided meditation and imagery.

Emotional Support

For most people, emotional support during a health crisis means turning to family and friends. It is also essential to have support from your primary health provider. The "Healing Connections" section of *Step Four* addresses the importance of social supports to promote health. If you do not have a strong support system, you may need to reach out to others in order to create one. There are many options open to you. You can contact a church or spiritual group, the hospital pastoral counseling office, general or health-oriented support groups, and organizations like Hospice.

Churches and spiritual groups have prayer circles, healing rituals and ceremonies, and members who will visit you in the hospital and at home following surgery. Hospital pastoral counseling offices usually serve Protestant, Catholic, and Jewish faiths, but they will provide you with support regardless of your religious affiliation. The Center for Attitudinal Healing, which offers free health-oriented support groups, also provides a free home and hospital visiting service. In and outside of the hospital, you have access to fee-charging psychotherapists and social workers.

Extended hospital stays and recovery periods may necessitate the use of a health care advocate who provides a very specific type of emotional support. Advocates help you address consumer health care issues when you are ill.

In the hospital, they can intercede on your behalf with a health provider, arrange special menus with nutritionists, request uninterrupted rest from the nursing staff, and deal with your insurance company. Outside the hospital, a health care advocate can accompany you to preparatory and follow-up health appointments, research treatment options, pick up prescribed medications, and help you with self-care issues like caring for a wound or incision.

Hospitals

Hospitals are in the business of making customers like you happy, and most hospitals will accommodate your desire to use alternative medicine and bodymind techniques to facilitate medical surgery and the recovery process. Screen prospective hospitals in advance of your admission to ensure their cooperation, and secure the necessary approvals to use alternative methods and techniques.

When you are in the hospital, develop a good relationship with the nursing staff because it can be difficult to use alternative methods and techniques without their cooperation and assistance. It is also important to have a good relationship with your surgeon and primary care doctor who can encourage hospital personnel to accommodate your special needs.

Some hospitals employ the services of a hospitalist, a general practice physician or internist who specializes in inpatient medicine and is responsible for managing the care of hospital patients. Most hospitals have patient or customer relations representatives to address your needs and concerns. Health care advocates can do all this and make decisions on your behalf in the event that you are incapacitated by complications resulting from surgery.

If hospitals are supposed to be places for getting well, why aren't they nicer places to be? Most hospitals are places from which people cannot wait to leave. Hopefully, this situation will change in the future. As a start, many hospitals now offer wellness programs with a holistic focus and provide alternative therapies such as biofeedback, massage, stress management, nutritional counseling, meditation, and yoga to patients on an outpatient basis. A handful of hospitals in the United States now also house alternative medicine clinics.

SUMMARY & FURTHER READING

Hospital Smarts, Kenneth Rothaus and Theodore Tyberg

After Surgery, Illness, or Trauma: 10 Practical Steps to Renewed Energy and Health, Regina Ryan

Consider using the following alternative methods and techniques to aid in the preparation for and recovery from medical surgery:

1. Herbs & Supplements

The Herbs of Life, Lesley Tierra, L.Ac., Herbalist

The Way of Herbs, Michael Tierra, L.Ac., O.M.D.

The Healing Power of Herbs, Michael Murray, N.D.

Healthy Healing, Linda Page, N.D., Ph.D.

Prescription for Nutritional Healing, James F. Balch, M.D. and Phyllis A. Balch, CNC

2. Aromatherapy

   The Aromatherapy Book, Applications and Inhalations, Jeanne Rose

   The Complete Book of Essential Oils and Aromatherapy, Valerie Ann Worwood

3. Guided Meditations & Imagery

   Guided Imagery for Self-Healing, Martin L. Rossman, M.D.

   Rituals of Healing: Using Imagery for Health and Wellness, Jeanne Achterberg, Barbara Dossey, and Leslie Kolkmeier

4. Music Therapy

   Sound Health, Steven Halpern

5. Positive Affirmations

   Healing Words for the Body, Mind and Spirit: 101 Words to Inspire and Affirm, Caren Goldman

6. Emotional Support

   The Support Group Sourcebook, Linda L. Klein

   Self-Help Groups for Coping With Crisis, M.A. Lieberman

CHAPTER 7

APPROACH DEATH & DYING
WITH A NEW VIEW

E very ancient spiritual tradition tells us that death is not the end. This seems difficult for us to believe because body, mind, and spirit have been so successfully separated from one another for the past four centuries. Eastern spiritual masters sometimes ask prospective students if they believe in life after death. For them, believing in life after death "alters the entire outlook on life and gives the believer a sense of personal responsibility and morality." In many ways, death and dying is the topic most relevant to illness. Our beliefs about death directly affect how we regard life and illness. A famous saying goes, "As soon as we're born, we're dead."

What is illness? Illness is a physical, emotional, and spiritual disharmony between you and nature or the eternal force. When you resist or oppose the flow of nature, illness results. Illness represents an imbalance between the heart and mind, the emergence of some unfinished business, or the completion of a life's work. It can occur for the purpose of learning, growth, love, awareness, compassion, or the resolution of karmic consequences. In this regard, illness is not a foreign invader but is indigenous to us, emerging from our own nature rather than from anything that exists outside of us. There is a positive aspect to every illness because it provides us with the opportunity to bring our attention to the underlying basis for the imbalance. In this way, bad habits or accidents are only symptoms of illness rather than the causes of it.

What is healing? Healing is the restoration of harmony between you and nature or the eternal force. When you no longer resist or oppose the flow of nature, healing results. Healing signifies the balance of the heart and mind, the resolution of unfinished business, or the completion of a life's work. It may manifest itself in the removal of disease from the body, a change in attitude or perception in the face of continuing or worsened incapacitation, or leaving the body behind in order to restore balance and harmony. Healing can also bring about learning, growth, love, awareness, compassion, or the resolution of karmic consequences. It results from a true understanding of the underlying nature of illness, not just an awareness of the symptoms of it.

In this expanded view, healing and wellness are not necessarily synonymous with physical health, and illness and disease are not necessarily synonymous with a lack of physical health. Illness begets suffering, which begets the evolution of the human soul, which begets the meaning of life. Every soul has a special purpose or sacred contract, which may be very different for those who find themselves in exactly the same circumstances. Healing is only realized through an understanding of man's indivisibility with nature and the purpose of the soul. Perfect healing always occurs in an environment of unconditional love.

A perception of healing that is dependent on finding external answers to external problems diminishes the efficacy of any medicine and possibility for true healing. A perception of healing that is dependent on a willingness to seek deeper meaning from the experience encourages the efficacy of treatment and possibility for true healing. The priority of any person who wishes to be healed is to awaken to the natural forces of his true nature rather than to be pre-occupied with achieving physical recovery. To do this is to discover the living presence within us that is not affected by time, space, or circumstance.

Your true nature may be best described as what you are meant to be but have yet to become. To awaken to the natural forces of your true nature is to understand the purpose of your soul. Your true nature also signifies an awareness of your humanness. In order to realize this, you must possess an awareness that lies beyond humanness. Awakening to the natural forces of your true nature and understanding the purpose of your soul ultimately restores the harmony and balance between you and nature.

Life, death, and healing are all one and the same; only the level of awareness changes. Eastern spiritual traditions approach life as preparation for death, which they regard as the beginning of another life. We separate life from death through our emotional attachments. If death is regarded as an avoidable enemy, an unavoidable inevitability, or as a means to escape life, life and death are separated from one another. Dedication to the exclusive goal of physical recovery over seeking harmony with nature or to a belief in a source of healing other than yourself also causes life and death to be separated from one another.

The separation of life from death and man from them both cause us to make protective attachments to these illusory states. When there is something to protect, the ego gets involved. When the focus is on protection rather than awakening or opening to life, the glory of life is overlooked altogether. The separation of life and death is synonymous with the separation of the heart and mind, placing us in a disharmonious position with nature before illness is ever man-ifested. *It is the separate attachment to life and death that does not allow true healing to take place*. It is important to be open to the possibility of life or death without expectation, to focus on the desire for inner truth, which is also universal truth.

This is a perspective many of us have difficulty under-standing because our society does not encourage us to regard life with such connectedness. We have learned to equate healing with physical recovery and to avoid loss at all costs—especially death. To avoid death is also to fear death. It is this fear of death and the attachment to ego that results from the separation of life from death.

To fear death is also to sometimes misuse technology to sustain life. This can be contrary to the flow of nature if it involves the delay of an inevitable healing that can only be realized through death. Science has made great inroads into prolonging life, and it is certainly advantageous to have more time to learn life lessons. It is important to ask, however, if the quality of life is improved by technological intervention and if there are still tasks to be accomplished or lessons to be learned. Sometimes, prolonging life is more about a fear of death and its unnatural postponement than a genuine desire to sustain life. This results in a diminishment of life rather than an enhancement of it.

How to transform a fear of death so it is inseparable from life is a difficult task. The concept of some continuation of life after death makes this transformation possible. A con-tinuation of life refers to the living presence, a conscious immortality or cosmic consciousness that continues after the body ceases to exist. Life after death can also refer to the physical rebirth of the human soul, known in Eastern reli-gions as reincarnation.

If death is not the end, it ceases to be an enemy. We are, therefore, more *in* the world than *of* the world, a concept written about in many religious scriptures including the Bible.

The ancient wisdom traditions, mystical heritages, and indigenous cultures have much in common in this regard. They all include a belief in the importance of awareness, intention, morality, love, wisdom, purpose, and service. They also refer to a visual one-pointedness, leading to states of luminosity and inner splendor. Although there are variances in the way these traditions describe the human experience and reach their spiritual goals, they are much more alike than they are different.

The more removed from the mysticism of the wisdom traditions and the original word of the great spiritual prophets, the basis for many of them, the greater the tendency we have, in the name of organized religion, to ignore or reject the basic universal truths. As we know, organized religion, a man-made creation, does not always reflect the benevolent laws of the universe.

The idea that souls move through many lifetimes for the purpose of learning and evolution is also held as a basic universal truth by many ancient wisdom traditions and heritages. Before its secularization, Christianity embraced more mystical notions like these as did Judaism. Tibetans, who have made spirituality their primary avocation, believe in many transitions: birth to death, death to rebirth, and dreaming, which they also regard as a transitional state. Some Tibetan teachers have jokingly said that they are more afraid of rebirth than death, suggesting not only a life after death but one that is superior to life in the physical world.

A few decades ago, the concept of rebirth or a continuation of life seemed absurd to most people. Today, the search for greater meaning in life has opened our minds to this esoteric concept. This concept is the basis for past life regression therapy, which allows people to remember experiences from previous lifetimes, helping them to resolve current problems. (See *Step Four*.) For many years, scientists have also studied the Near Death Experience (NDE) and report that people recount the same journey to an afterlife and back to consciousness in remarkable detail.

A mystical view of life renders death a mere transition from one state of being to the next. All endings including death have a beginning, and all beginnings have an ending. With this belief, there is no loss.

First-century Roman emperor and philosopher Marcus Aurelius said in his *Meditations*, "You are a little soul carrying around a corpse." If our bodies are like a set of clothes that we shed from lifetime to lifetime, then death is not an end but a door through which our souls pass over and over again. Death is life and life is death from this perspective. They are truly inseparable. No longer an enemy to be feared or fought against or an object of desire to put us out of our misery, death is neither friend nor foe.

If we accept this understanding of life and death, we are liberated from the attachment to life and the struggle to hang onto it. Whether the healing process entails life or death can be received with love and detachment. The goal of healing can become the pursuit of balance and harmony with the forces of nature over the struggle for physical recovery or to stay alive.

The route to achieving balance and harmony is through a surrender to unconditional love. A surrender to unconditional love also allows life and death to merge into one and provides insight into the human experience in which a higher purpose is perceived in every circumstance. In this context, to surrender does not mean to give up but to have loving trust toward something.

True healing occurs in an atmosphere of unconditional love and becomes the ultimate freedom. An atmosphere of unconditional love arises from a meditative mind and a generous spirit, which is achieved by quieting the mind and opening the heart. To quiet the mind and open the heart is to increase awareness through the development of an inner life, the connection of the soul to the creative part of the universe and a portal to universal truth and healing. This connection opens us to an infinite capacity for love and an understanding of the meaning in life. It is also the living presence within us that is not affected by time, space, or circumstance. It is our true nature.

The development of an inner life automatically changes our outer view. The inward journey provides the seeker with transcendent and luminous moments of vision, which are not accessible from outside or worldly sources. With regular practice, it leads to what-is-often-described-as a nothingness or emptiness that goes beyond mere words, actions, and the ego of the mind. The inward journey elevates and transports us from the bottom of the abyss to a state of bliss.

The development of an inner life is the key to discovering your true nature and the foundation of all spiritual traditions. An inner life can be developed through some form of daily inward-focused discipline or practice, whether it is through the prayer of Christianity or Judaism, the vision quest of shamanic tradition, or the meditation, prostrations, chanting, and visualizations of Eastern spiritual traditions. An inner life can also be developed through simple contemplation.

True spiritual traditions withstand the scrutiny of their participants. No matter how ancient a spiritual tradition is, no spiritual journey is truly authentic unless it is thoroughly questioned and totally experienced in the heart and mind of the seeker. An authentic spiritual journey is not like an article of clothing you put on simply when it suits you. It is not based on how well the scriptures are quoted or how many meditation retreats have been attended. A spiritual journey becomes authentic when the experience of it is fully recognized and lived. Only when the seeker is truly sincere will answers follow.

Seekers must find their own path to spiritual awareness— one that can only be taken alone. This inevitably involves the experience of solitude. Solitude is not synonymous with loneliness. Loneliness refers to the neediness of the ego. Solitude creates the opportunity to join with the higher forces in the universe. In solitude, you are never alone, quite the opposite. The solitude of contemplative practice or an inner life helps us to understand that life as we know it on the surface is not all there is. Through this expanded awareness and knowledge lies true healing.

Why should we change our view about death and dying after a lifetime of regarding it as an object of fear and avoidance, you might ask? There is absolutely nothing to lose and much to gain by doing so. Pascal's Wager is named after a seventeenth-century French scientist who began to believe in God as a result of a mystical experience. It postulates that you lose nothing by believing in a higher power and stand to gain everything if the existence of a higher power turns out to be true. Not only is there no disadvantage to believing in life after death, but it also eliminates the fear of death and eases human suffering.

Believing in the universality of all sentient beings gives meaning to senseless acts such as the death of a child, a crippling accident, an incurable illness, and even murder. It explains why bad things happen to good people and helps us forgive our worst enemies. A belief in life after death allows for the possibility of infinite reunion with the people we love. It signifies inescapable consequences for every thought, word, and deed—what is termed fate or destiny and known in Eastern cultures as karma.

It is no coincidence that unexplainable tragedies, along with aging, have the power to convert limited faith into a steadfast belief in some form of an afterlife. This is not desperation; it is realization.

Imagine how different our behavior toward one another would be if we understood that the consequences of our actions or inactions followed us into future lifetimes. Do we isolate people from us who are suffering? Do we hurt others because we are hurting? Do we create harm through a disregard for our environment? The response to our own suffering and the suffering of others will determine future lessons we will face. Each of us has a destiny that we have created for ourselves through our past thoughts, words, and deeds.

A belief in life after death demands greater respect for destiny and the synchronicity of life. This respect tells us that there are no accidents in life and that serendipitous experience is not mere coincidence. Greater value is also placed on our innate ability to intuit a higher purpose for our experiences.

With this understanding comes the knowledge that destiny does not preclude free will or imply helplessness. In fact, destiny signifies *helpfulness* because it provides us with the knowledge and experience from which we can learn, grow, evolve, and elevate the soul. "You reap what you sow," from Galatians in the *Holy Bible,* or the popular saying "what goes around comes around" may have more meaning and significance in our lives than we ever imagined possible.

When the concept of rebirth is understood, the infrastructure of everyday life, along with the artifice of our egos, becomes superfluous, much like imaginary prison walls that surround us. It becomes clear that we are judged on metaphysical terms for our humanity rather than on our acquisitions of money, possessions, power, fame, or control. A growing disenchantment with worldly pursuits marks the need to initiate an inner search for greater meaning in life—a search for our humanity.

When the physical body dies, the body of ego or self-image is relinquished. The body of spirit is still vibrant and alive. Instead of death taking us to another place, our souls simply understand and remember where they always were as a continuation of our cosmic consciousness.

Why not believe that life is a transitory stage rather than the end of existence? What purpose does a belief like this serve except to create hope for us all? If life and death were viewed in this way, we would celebrate death with the same promise and reverence that we use to celebrate life.

Practical Considerations

Although 70% of respondents said in a recent poll that they want to die at home, in reality, 75% of deaths occur in medical institutions. It is estimated that almost 50% of deaths involve people who die in pain and are surrounded by strangers, three out of five medical doctors knowing their clients for less than one week. Many people complain that their wishes for medical treatment are disregarded or ignored. Costs for dying are high and approximate $1,000 per day in a hospital, $1,000 per week in a nursing home, $700 per week for hospice care. These statistics demonstrate that you must take precautions to avoid such disastrous possibilities.

There are several practical steps you can initiate if you are faced with the prospect of death and even if you are not. Let your wishes be known in the form of a living will, living trust, or advance health care directive. These legal documents spell out the extent to which you want your life prolonged or sustained with medical intervention and under what circumstances you want to be resuscitated from cardiac or respiratory arrest. They can also outline your wishes for the disposition of your body by burial or cremation and can detail special funeral or memorial requests. Along with a health care power of attorney, a health care advocate can be designated in these documents to make decisions on your behalf if you are incapacitated and to ensure that your wishes are carried out.

By incorporating advance health care directives and the selection of an advocate in a legal document, you can exercise choice in these matters before they become a complicated or controversial legal issue. Make sure that your living will, living trust, or advance health care directive follows state guidelines so that it will be legally upheld. All legal and financial documents regarding your wishes should be kept together in a secure place, and family, friends, an attorney, or your advocate should be advised of their location.

Guides to executing these documents can be found at Nolo Press at (800) 728–3555 or www.nolo.com and Aging With Dignity at (850) 681–2010 or www.agingwithdignity. org. You can also register your living will or advance health care directive with the corporate-sponsored U.S. Living Will Registry at (800) 548–9455 or www.uslivingwillregistry.com.

Familiarize yourself with the benefits your health insurance policy pays for terminal care. Private health insurance policies vary significantly in their coverage of home health care, hospice services, prescription drugs, and other life-support services. If you have limited coverage for these services, you may want to buy a supplemental policy.

Medicare, which covers more than 80% of people who are facing death, does not pay benefits for every health expense. If you are eligible for Medicare, you may want to buy a Medigap policy for expenses Medicare does not cover. You can also purchase long-term health insurance for expenses not covered by Medicare and policies to cover chronic care, nonmedical services, and nursing homes.

There are many organizations that help people prepare for death. The traditional hospice movement, although limited in its capacity to transform the view of death and dying, provides valuable physical, emotional, and spiritual support for people in transition from this lifetime. In order to have hospice care covered by health insurance, two medical doctors are required to verify that the insured has six months or less to live. Hospice centers are located throughout the world. Contact the National Hospice & Palliative Care Organization at (800) 658–8898.

The Zen Hospice Project in San Francisco combines traditional hospice service with Buddhist traditions in an effort to create a more meaningful death experience. Contact the Project at (415) 863–2910. Other alternatives to the traditional approach to death and dying include Partnership for Caring at (800) 989–9455, Death With Dignity National Center at (202) 969–1669, and M.I.S.S. Foundation at (623) 979–1000. For a list of international death, dying, and bereavement workshops with an alternative approach, contact the Externalization Workshops at (413) 268–7342.

The National Mental Health Association at (800) 969–6642 offers information and a guide to overcoming grief. Compassionate Friends at (877) 969–0010 and In Loving Memory at (703) 435–3111 (Fax) offers assistance to grieving parents. Hospitals, community social services, and privately funded groups offer support for the dying. Consult your library for a list of resources in your community. Some groups do not advertise, so it is wise to ask around.

People with terminal illness sometimes consider the option of physician-assisted suicide or euthanasia, although this procedure is still very controversial. The Oregon-based Hemlock Society provides consumer information on the right to die. Its founder and former executive director Derek Humphry published a book titled *Final Exit: The Practicalities of Self-deliverance and Assisted Suicide for the Dying*. Oregon is currently the only state with legalized physician-assisted suicide, although other states such as Hawaii are considering similar legislation. Contact the National Hemlock Society at (800) 247–7421.

SUMMARY & FURTHER READING

Who Dies?, Stephen Levine

The Tibetan Book of Living and Dying,
   Sogyal Rinpoche

1. Execute a living will, trust, or health care directive that clearly outlines your medical and burial wishes.

2. Familiarize yourself with the health benefits your insurer pays for terminal care, and supplement your policy if necessary.

3. Make sure that your family, friends, attorney, and/or health care advocate know your wishes and have access to the appropriate legal documents.

4. Utilize support services for death and dying such as hospice that are located in your community.

CHAPTER 8

CONCLUSION

Healing means different things to different people and does not exclusively pertain to physical recovery. Some people experience healing from a new attitude, insight into an unresolved issue, a gesture of kindness, the birth of a child, an act of self-discovery, a moment of grace, or even death. It is more important to cultivate health than to eliminate illness. With this as our goal, we must be willing to accept a broader vision of what it means to be healed.

A healing journey involves many layers of investigation and intervention. Interventions such as those described in the six-step plan facilitate change and lead to true healing, especially if you are willing to assume an active role in the process. Doing nothing is also an intervention if its purpose is to allow the body to rest from treatment or to allow previous interventions the time to work

It is important to remember that motivations, intentions, and expectations matter, yours and those belonging to the people who are treating you. All alternative medicine is not good and must be approached with a consumer's caution and good judgment. Alternative medicine is also highly individualized, requiring a great deal of patience and self-reliance in order to be fully understood and used wisely. It is important to do what you can and not feel terrible about what you cannot do. Using one alternative practice or medicine well is better than using many alternative practices or medicines poorly.

As a responsible health care consumer, you are obliged to do three things when confronted with a health crisis:

- *see*—keep events in perspective by understanding that illness exists to serve learning, not to punish.

- *explore and change*—look for answers and change what can be changed.

- *surrender*—trust what is and let go of what is not.

In the final analysis, when reliance on external interventions is exhausted, you must eventually face yourself. In this moment, it seems that nothing more can be done; you feel abandoned and the most alone. When this happens, it may be helpful to approach your problems with the understanding that *it is not what happens to you, but how you respond to what happens to you that truly matters.* How you play the hand is far more important than what cards you are dealt.

Although there is an obligation to look for answers in the presence of adversity, sometimes the answer is to know when to let go of the need for explanation because it is not always possible to know why something has happened. We must begin to learn to embrace and value the mystical and inexplicable in our lives. The physicist Albert Einstein said, "The most beautiful thing we can experience is the mysterious." If we can do this, we will realize that illness is an exceptional opportunity for change and growth.

We must also let go of the need for perfection because it is not always possible to function so perfectly that we can avoid adversity altogether. No amount of knowledge, action, or awareness will stop life from throwing curves. Musician John Lennon's song lyric states, "Life is just what happens to you while you're busy making other plans."

It is a Western misconception that being blessed is synonymous with material success, fame, or good fortune. The ability to learn, grow, and find happiness in misfortune is not only the greater challenge but the greater blessing. Profound life lessons are offered to us in the most painful moments and the opportunity for personal growth and transformation is always created through adversity.

The person who regards difficult life circumstances as a gift is the person who is truly blessed. This is the path that ultimately leads to true healing. As Lao Tzu said so eloquently in the *Tao Te Ching*, "A person will get well when he is tired of being sick."

A recipe by an unknown author:

Take twelve whole months,
Clean them thoroughly of all bitterness, rumors, hate and
  jealousy (make them as fresh and clean as possible)
Now cut each month into 28, 30, or 31 different parts.
But don't make up the whole batch at once . . .
Instead prepare it "one day at a time."
Mix well each day with:
  one part Faith
  one part Patience
  one part Courage
  one part Work,
Add one part each of Hope, Honesty,
  Generosity and Kindness

Blend with:
  one part Prayer
  one part Meditation
  at least one Good Deed
Season the whole with a dash of Good Spirit,
  a sprinkle of Fun,
A pinch of Play and a cupful of Good Humor.
Pour all of this into a vessel of Love.
Cook thoroughly over radiant Joy.
Garnish with Smiles.
And serve with Quietness, Unselfishness and Good
  Cheer...
And you are bound to make a Life of Happiness and Peace.

And Good Health!

SUMMARY

The *10 Keys to Successfully Using Alternative Medicine* are:

1. Approach alternative medicine with a different attitude and expectation. Be willing to assume responsibility for your care by becoming more empowered in the healing process.

2. Alternative medicine is not a substitute for a healthy lifestyle nor is it a panacea for personal or societal stress.

3. There is no magic bullet in any healing process and no guarantee of health from any external intervention. Healing is an internal process and a state of mind.

4. All aspects of wellness—physical, emotional, spiritual—must be in balance and harmony in order for true healing to take place.

5. To ensure the safe use of alternative medicine: educate yourself about your options, consult with qualified practitioners to determine your particular health care needs, and make lifestyle and other changes gradually.

6. The key to healing is self-empowerment, which includes your full and active participation in the health care process and an ability to surrender to the experience.

7. Self-empowerment is achieved by increasing awareness.

8. Increased awareness is facilitated by the development of an inner life.

9. The development of an inner life is accomplished by simplifying your life, surrounding yourself with silence, and learning to use the breath.

10. Learning to use the breath in a regular inner practice or discipline is the most powerful instrument or tool to increase awareness and promote true healing.

PROFESSIONAL ASSOCIATIONS & ORGANIZATIONS

Please note: *Phone numbers are constantly subject to change. Please consult the appropriate directory if the number listed below is no longer in service.*

Acupuncture

Acupuncture & Oriental Medicine Alliance (253) 851–6896

American Academy of Medical Acupuncture (323) 937–5514

American Association of Oriental Medicine (301) 941–1064 or (888) 500–7999

National Certification Commission for Acupuncture and Oriental Medicine (703) 548–9004

Aikido

Aikido Association of America (773) 525–3141

International Directory Aikido Schools (800) 445–2454

Alternative Medicine—General

American Association for Health Freedom (800) 230–2762

American Board of Holistic Medicine (808) 572–4616

American Holistic Health Association (714) 779–6152

American Holistic Medical Association (505) 292–7788

American Holistic Nurses Association (800) 278–2462

American Holistic Veterinary Medical Association
(410) 569–0795

Complementary-Alternative Medical Association
(404) 284–7592

Holistic Dental Association (970) 259–1091

National Center for Complementary and Alternative Medicine
(NIH) (301) 519–3153 or (888) 644–6226

National Wellness Institute (715) 342–2969 or
(800) 243–8694

National Women's Health Network (202) 347–1140

Society of Behavioral Medicine (608) 827–7267

Alternative Medicine—Miscellaneous

American Academy of Anti-Aging Medicine (773) 528–4333

American Academy of Pain Management (209) 533–9744

American Board of Chelation Therapy (800) 356–2228

Association for Applied Psychophysiology and Biofeedback
(303) 422–8436 or (800) 477–8892

Biofeedback Certification Institute of America (303) 420–2902

Institute of Noetic Sciences (707) 775–3500

International Association for Colon Hydrotherapy
(210) 366–2888

International Association for Oxygen Therapy (208) 448–2504

Midwives' Alliance of North America (888) 923–6262

Alternative Medicine Clinics (within hospitals)
Note: Many local hospitals now offer wellness programs on an outpatient basis.

Alliance Institute for Integrative Medicine, Health Alliance of
Greater Cincinnati, Cincinnati, Ohio, (513) 791–5521

Alternative Medicine Clinic, Fairview-University Medicine
Center, Minneapolis, Minnesota, (612) 672–6000

Center for Complementary Medicine, University of Pittsburgh Medical Center, Pittsburgh, Pennsylvania, (412) 647–3555 or (800) 533–8762

Department of Complementary Medicine Services Clinic, New York Presbyterian Hospital, New York, New York, (212) 342–0101

Institute for Health and Healing, California Pacific Medical Center, San Francisco, California, (415) 600–3660

Integrative Medicine Clinic, University of Arizona Health Sciences Center, Tucson, Arizona, (520) 626–7222

Mind/Body Medical Clinic and Institute, Beth Israel Deaconess Medical Center, Boston, Massachusetts, (617) 991–0102 or (866) 509–0732

Stress Reduction Clinic, University of Massachusetts Medical Center, Worcester, Massachusetts, (508) 856–2656

Aromatherapy

Association of Medical Aromatherapists, 11 Park Circus, Glasgow, UK, 684 8NF, 0141–332–4924

National Association for Holistic Aromatherapy (206) 547–2164 or (888) 275–6242

Pacific Institute of Aromatherapy (415) 479–9121

Attitudinal Healing

Center for Attitudinal Healing (415) 331–6161

Progoff Intensive Journal® Workshops (800) 221–5844

Ayurveda

American Association of Ayurvedic Sciences (425) 453–8022 (medical clinic)

Ayurveda Holistic Center and School of Ayurvedic Science (800) 452–1798

Ayurvedic Institute (505) 291–9698

Chopra Center for Well Being (888) 424–6772

College of Maharishi Ayurveda (800) 369–6480 (instruction only)

Maharishi Ayurveda Medical Centers:

Albuquerque, New Mexico (800) 811–0550

Bethesda, Maryland (301) 770–5690

Dallas, Texas (888) 259–9915

Fairfield, Iowa (800) 248–9050

Lancaster, Massachusetts (877) 890–8600

Bodywork—Miscellaneous

American Society for the Alexander Technique (413) 584–2359 or (800) 473–0620

Association for Meridian Energy Therapies, 18 Marlow Avenue, Eastbourne, East Sussex, BN22 8SJ, UK, +44–132–3729666

Federation of Therapeutic Massage, Bodywork and Somatic Practice Organizations (847) 864–0123

Hellerwork International (800) 392–3900

International Association of Reiki Professionals (603) 881–8838

International Nurses Association Complementary Therapists (504) 893–8002

National Association of Myofascial Trigger Point Therapists (800) 845–3454

Nurse Healers-Professional Associates International (801) 273–3399

Rolf Institute (303) 449–5903

Trager Association (216) 896–9383

Chiropractic Medicine

American Chiropractic Association (703) 243–2593 or (800) 986–4636

International Chiropractors Association (703) 528–5000 or (800) 423–4690

International College of Applied Kinesiology (913) 384–5336

Consumer Advocacy Groups

Campaign for Environmentally Responsible Health Care (202) 234–9121

Center for Medical Consumers (212) 674–7105

Citizen's Council on Health Care (651) 646–8935

Citizens for Health (202) 483–4344

Committee for Freedom of Choice in Medicine (800) 227–4473 or (619) 429–8200

Consumer's Union (914) 378–2000

National Women's Health Network (202) 628–7814

Public Citizen Health Research Group (202) 588–1000

Death & Dying

Compassionate Friends (630) 990–0010 or (877) 969–0010

Death With Dignity National Center (202) 969–1669

Externalization Workshops (413) 268–7342

In Loving Memory (703) 435–3111 (Fax)

M.I.S.S. Foundation (623) 979–1000

National Hemlock Society (800) 247–7421

National Hospice & Palliative Care Organization (703) 837–1500 or (800) 658–8898

National Mental Health Association (800) 969–6642

Partnership for Caring (202) 296–8071 or (800) 989–9455

Zen Hospice Project (415) 863–2910

Energy Medicine

International Society for the Study of Subtle Energies and Energy Medicine (303) 425–4625

Environmental Medicine

American Academy of Environmental Medicine (316) 684–5500

Environmental Illness Society of Canada (613) 728–9493

International Society for Environmental Illness in Germany at +40–641–99–41450

Feldenkrais Method

Feldenkrais Guild of North America (800) 775–2118

Feng Shui

Feng Shui Directory of Consultants (434) 973–7223 or (800) 443–5894

Yun Lin Temple (510) 841–2347

Guided Imagery

Academy for Guided Imagery (800) 726–2070

International Imagery Association (914) 476–0781

Herbal/Plant Medicine

American Association of Naturopathic Physicians (866) 538–2267

American Botanical Council (512) 926–4900

American Herbalists Guild (770) 751–6021

American Horticulture Therapy Association (800) 634–1603

Bach Flower Essences International Education Program (800) 334–0843

Dr. Edward Bach Centre, Mount Vernon, Baker's Lane, Sotwell, Oxon, OX10–0PZ, UK, 44(0)1491–834678

Herb Research Foundation (303) 449–2265

International Register of Herbalists and Aromatherapists, 32 King Edward Road, Swansea, UK SA1 4LL

World Wide Essence Society (978) 369–8454

Homeopathy

Homeopathic Academy of Naturopathic Physicians (208) 336–9242

International Register of Homeopathic Practitioners, 32 King Edward Road, Swansea, UK SA1 4LL

National Center for Homeopathy (703) 548–7790

Humor Therapy

American Association for Therapeutic Humor (602) 995–1454

Laughter Heals Foundation (818) 990–2019

Laughter Therapy Foundation, Box 827, Monterey, California, 93942

Hypnosis

American Society of Clinical Hypnosis (630) 980–4740

International Medical and Dental Hypnotherapy Association (800) 257–5467

Milton H. Erickson Foundation (602) 956–6196

National Guild of Hypnotists (603) 429–9438

Magnet Therapy

Bio-Electro-Magnetics Institute (775) 827–9099

International Foundation of Bio-Magnetics (520) 751–7751

Massage Therapy

American Academy of Reflexology (818) 841–7741

American Massage Therapy Association (847) 864–0123

American Organization for Bodywork Therapies of Asia
(856) 782–1616

American Oriental Bodywork Therapy Association
(856) 782–1616

Associated Bodywork and Massage Professionals
(800) 458–2267

International Institute of Reflexology (727) 343–4811

International Massage Association (540) 351–0800

National Certification for Therapeutic Massage and Bodywork
(800) 296–0664

Reflexology Association of America (508) 364–4234

Medical Qigong

International Institute of Medical Qigong (831) 646–9399

National Qigong Association (218) 365–6330

World Society of Medical Qigong, 9 Hepingjie Beikou,
Chaoyang District, Beijing 100013, People's Republic of
China, +86–1–4211591

Meditation

Insight Meditation:

Inquiring Mind, P.O. Box 9999, North Berkeley, CA 94709

Insight Meditation Society (978) 355–4378

Transcendental Meditation®:

Transcendental Meditation Center (626) 799–1821

Transcendental Meditation Program (888) 532–7686

Music/Sound/Light Therapy

American Association for Music Therapy (301) 589–3300

Society for Light Treatment and Biological Rhythms
(415) 751–2758 (Fax)

Naturopathy

American Association of Naturopathic Physicians
(202) 895–1392 or (866) 538–2267
American Naturopathic Medical Association (702) 897–7053
Homeopathic Academy of Naturopathic Physicians
(208) 336–9242

Nutrition

American Association of Nutritional Consultants
(888) 828–2262
American Dietetic Association (800) 366–1655
Nutrition Education Association (713) 665–2946
Society of Certified Nutritionists (800) 342–8037

Orthomolecular Medicine

Linus Pauling Institute (541) 737–5075

Osteopathic Medicine & Craniosacral Therapy

American Academy of Osteopathy (317) 879–1881
American Osteopathic Assocation (800) 621–1773
Upledger Institute (561) 622–4334

Polarity Therapy

American Polarity Therapy Association (303) 545–2080

Psychotherapy

American Association for Marriage and Family Therapy
(202) 452–0109
American Counseling Association (703) 823–9800 or
(800) 347–6647
American Psychiatric Association (703) 907–7300

American Psychological Association (202) 336–5500 or
   (800) 374–2721

Association for Humanistic Psychology (510) 769–6495

Association for Transpersonal Psychology (650) 424–8764

International Association of Counselors and Therapists
   (941) 498–9710

International Somatic Movement Education and Therapy
   Association (212) 229–7666

National Association of Social Workers (202) 408–8600

Society for Spirituality and Social Work (607) 777–4603

U.S. Association for Body Psychotherapy (202) 446–1619

Qigong

American Foundation of Traditional Chinese Medicine
   (415) 392–7002

East West Academy of Health Arts (415) 788–2227

National Qigong Association (218) 365–6330

Qigong Institute (650) 323–1221

Regression Therapy

Association for Past-Life Research and Therapies
   (909) 784–1570

Milton H. Erickson Foundation (602) 956–6196

Spiritual Healing

Casa de Dom Ignacio (House of St. Ignatius Loyola),
   Abadiania, Brazil, +55–62–343–1254 (Fax)

National Federation of Spiritual Healers, Old Manor Farm
   Studio, Church Street, Sunbury-on-Thames, Middlesex,
   UK, TW16 6RG, +44–845–1232777

Tai Chi

American Foundation of Traditional Chinese Medicine
(415) 956–3030

Tibetan Medicine

Chakpori Institute, 151–31 88th Street, Box 2D,
Howard Beach, NY 11414, (718) 641–7323

Yoga

American Yoga Association (941) 927–4977

Yoga Alliance (877) 964–2255

Yoga Research and Education Center (530) 474–5700

INTERNET RESOURCES

Please note: *Here is a small sampling of the thousands of websites on alternative medicine. Many of the organizations listed in Appendix A also maintain websites. Remember to consider the source and reasonableness of the information and exercise extreme caution before buying any products online. The Federal Trade Commission maintains a listing of recommended health websites at www.ftc.gov.*

Acupuncture.com
acupuncture.com

Aging with Dignity
www.agingwithdignity.org

Alternative Health News Online
www.altmedicine.com

Alternative Medicine
www.pitt.edu/~cbw/altm.html

Alternative Medicine Directory
www.altmedicine.net

Alternative Medicine Magazine
www.alternativemedicine.com

Anti-Aging Medicine
www.worldhealth.net

Ask Dr. Weil
www.drweil.com

Blue Shield of California
www.mylifepath.com

Body & Soul Magazine
www.bodyandsoulmag.com

Chakpori Institute (Tibetan Medicine)
www.tibetanmedicine.com

Chinese Herb Database
www.chinaginseng.com

Commonweal
www.commonweal.org

East West School of Herbology
www.planetherbs.com

Emotional Healing Resources
www.holisticmed.com/www/psychology.html

Esalen Retreat Center
www.esalen.org

Externalization Workshops
www.externalizationworkshops.com

Feng Shui Directory
www.fengshuidirectory.com

Griefnet
rivendell.org

Health and Healing News
www.hhnews.com

HealthWorld Online
www.healthy.net

Homeopathic Educational Services
www.homeopathic.com

Illustrated Herbal Encyclopedia
www.canoe.ca/HealthHerbal/home.html

Intuition Network
www.intuition.org

Laughter Heals Foundation
www.laughterheals.com

Living and Raw Foods Community
www.living-foods.com

National Center for Complementary and Alternative
Medicine
www.nccam.nih.gov

New Age Web Works
www.newageinfo.com

New Hope Natural Media Online
www.newhope.com

Omega Institute
www.eomega.org

Pharminfonet
www.pharminfo.com

Prevention Magazine
www.healthyideas.com

Prevention Medicine Research Institute
www.pmri.org

Share Guide
www.shareguide.com

Spirit Rock Meditation Center
www.spiritrock.org

Tai Chi
www.thetaichisite.com

U.S. Association for Body Psychotherapy
www.usabp.org

Yoga Journal Magazine
www.yogajournal.com

Six-Step Workbook

STEP ONE
Assess Your Lifestyle
A Precondition to Alternative Medicine Treatment

1. Diet _____

   _____

2. Exercise _____

   _____

3. Rest and Relaxation _____
   a. Regular Quiet Time _____
   b. Use the Breath _____
   c. Improve Sleep _____

4. Environment _____

   _____

5. Other _____

   _____

Notes: _____

_____

_____

STEP TWO
Balance Your Space
"External Energy Work"

Consult an external energetic specialist about environmental balance.

1. Feng Shui _____

_____

_____

_____

_____

2. Vastu Shastra _____

_____

_____

_____

_____

3. Other_____

_____

_____

_____

_____

Notes: _____

_____

_____

_____

STEP THREE
Balance Your Energy
"Internal Energy Work"

Choose a comprehensive medicine system to incorporate into your healing program.

1. Chinese medicine _____

_____

_____

2. Homeopathy_____

_____

_____

3. Ayurveda_____

_____

_____

4. Naturopathy _____

_____

_____

5. Other_____

_____

_____

Notes: _____

_____

_____

_____

STEP FOUR
Balance Your Mind
Mind Work"

Choose appropriate mindwork tools to incorporate into your healing program.

1. Immune-Building Characteristics_____

   _____

2. A Healing Attitude_____

   _____

3. Hypnosis and Guided Imagery _____

   _____

4. Regression Therapy _____

   _____

5. Healing Connections_____

   _____

6. Humor_____

   _____

7. Other_____

   _____

Notes: _____

_____

_____

_____

STEP FIVE
Balance Your Body
"Body Work"

Choose appropriate bodywork therapies to incorporate into your healing program:

1. Massage Therapy _____

_____

2. Craniosacral Therapy _____

_____

3. Feldenkrais Method _____

_____

4. Polarity Therapy _____

_____

5. Medical Qigong _____

_____

6. Other _____

_____

_____

Notes: _____

_____

_____

_____

STEP SIX
Prevent Future Imbalance
"Soul Work"

Initiate the regular practice of an inward discipline.

1. Meditation _____

   _____

   _____

2. Yoga_____

   _____

   _____

3. Tai Chi_____

   _____

   _____

4. Qigong _____

   _____

   _____

5. Other_____

   _____

   _____

Notes: _____

_____

_____

_____

Alternative Practitioners

Name: _____

Contact: _____

Speciality: _____

Notes: _____

_____

Name: _____

Contact: _____

Speciality: _____

Notes: _____

_____

Name: _____

Contact: _____

Speciality: _____

Notes: _____

_____

Name: _____

Contact: _____

Speciality: _____

Notes: _____

_____

Alternative Practitioners

Name: _____

Contact: _____

Speciality: _____

Notes: _____

_____

Name: _____

Contact: _____

Speciality: _____

Notes: _____

_____

Name: _____

Contact: _____

Speciality: _____

Notes: _____

_____

Name: _____

Contact: _____

Speciality: _____

Notes: _____

_____

Psychologists

Name: _____

Contact: _____

Speciality: _____

Notes: _____

_____

Name: _____

Contact: _____

Speciality: _____

Notes: _____

_____

Name: _____

Contact: _____

Speciality: _____

Notes: _____

_____

Name: _____

Contact: _____

Speciality: _____

Notes: _____

_____

Psychologists

Name: _____

Contact: _____

Speciality: _____

Notes: _____

_____

Name: _____

Contact: _____

Speciality: _____

Notes: _____

_____

Name: _____

Contact: _____

Speciality: _____

Notes: _____

_____

Name: _____

Contact: _____

Speciality: _____

Notes: _____

_____

Herbalists

Name: _____

Contact: _____

Speciality: _____

Notes: _____

_____

Name: _____

Contact: _____

Speciality: _____

Notes: _____

_____

Name: _____

Contact: _____

Speciality: _____

Notes: _____

_____

Name: _____

Contact: _____

Speciality: _____

Notes: _____

_____

Herbalists

Name: _____

Contact: _____

Speciality: _____

Notes: _____

_____

Name: _____

Contact: _____

Speciality: _____

Notes: _____

_____

Name: _____

Contact: _____

Speciality: _____

Notes: _____

_____

Name: _____

Contact: _____

Speciality: _____

Notes: _____

_____

BIBLIOGRAPHY

Please note: *For purposes of brevity, the many studies referred to in the guide are not cited. They can be found through the government agency that conducted the study or through the National Library of Medicine search engine PubMed® at* www.ncbi.nlm.nih.gov/PubMed/.

Agricultural Marketing Service. *National Organic Standards.* Washington, D.C.: U.S. Department of Agriculture, April 21, 2002.

Airola, Paavo. *Are You Confused?* Phoenix, Arizona: Health Plus, 1971.

Allione, Tsultrim. "Feeding the Demons: Relaxing Dualism." Speech presented at the 14th International Transpersonal Conference, Santa Clara, California, June 11, 1995.

American Bible Society. *Holy Bible: New Revised Standard Version.* New York: American Bible Society, 1989.

American Psychiatric Association. *Diagnostic and Statistical Manual of Mental Disorders.* 4th ed. Washington, D.C.: American Psychiatric Association, 1994.

Aurelius, Marcus. *The Meditations.* Translated by Gregory Hays. New York: The Modern Library, 2002.

Batmanghelidj, Fereydoon. *Your Body's Many Cries for Water.* Vienna, VA: Global Health Solutions, 1995.

Beinfield, Harriet, and Efrem Korngold. *Between Heaven And Earth, A Guide To Chinese Medicine.* New York: Ballantine Books, 1991.

Benson, Herbert, M.D. *Timeless Healing—the power and biology of belief.* New York: Simon and Schuster, 1997.

Braunwald, Eugene, et al. *Harrison's Principles of Internal Medicine.* 15th ed. New York: McGraw-Hill Professional, 2001.

Burton Goldberg Group. *Alternative Medicine.* Fife, Washington: Future Medicine, 1995.

California Department of Consumers Affairs. *Professional Therapy Never Includes Sex.* Sacramento, California, 2002.

Carrico, Mara. *Yoga Basics.* New York: Henry Holt and Company, Inc., 1997.

Chah, Venerable Ajaan. *Living Dhamma.* Thailand: The Sangha, Bung Wai Forest Monastery, 1992.

Clark, Hulda Regehr. *The Cure For All Disease.* San Diego, California: ProMotion Publishing, 1995.

Corliss, Richard, "The Power of Yoga," *Time,* April 23, 2001.

Cousins, Norman. *Anatomy of an Illness.* New York: W.W. Norton & Company, 1979.

Cox, Kathleen. *Vastu Living.* New York: Marlowe & Company, 2000.

Cummings, Stephen, and Dana Ullman. *Everybody's Guide to Homeopathic Medicines.* Los Angeles: Jeremy P. Tarcher, Inc., 1991.

Daryai Lal Kapur. *Call Of The Great Master.* Punjab, India: Radha Soami Satsang Beas, 1964.

Dement, William C., and Christopher Vaughan. *The Promise of Sleep.* New York: Dell Books, 2000.

Dreher, Henry. *The Immune Power Personality.* New York: Penguin Group, 1996.

Easwaran, Eknath. *Seeing With The Eyes Of Love.* Tomales, California: Nilgiri Press, 1996.

Flegal, Katherine M., et al. "Prevalence and Trends in Obesity Among U.S. Adults, 1999–2000." *Journal of American Medical Association* 288 (October 9, 2002): 1723–27.

Foodborne Active Diseases Surveillance Network. Morbidity and Mortality Weekly Report. *Preliminary FoodNet Data on the Incidence of Foodborne Illnesses—Selected Sites, United States, 2002.* Washington, D.C.: Centers for Disease Control and Prevention, April 18, 2003.

Freud, Sigmund. *Wit and Its Relation to the Unconscious.* New York: Moffat, Yard & Co., 1916.

Healthnotes® Online. Herb and remedy fact sheets [database online]. Portland, Oregon: Healthnotes, Inc. Available from http://www.healthnotes.com; INTERNET.

Hendler, Sheldon Saul. *The Oxygen Breakthrough: 30 days to an illness free life.* New York: Pocket Books, 1990.

Hippocrene Books. *Hippocrates.* Translated by W.H.S. Jones. Cambridge, MA: Harvard University Press, 1923.

Kastner, Mark, and Hugh Burroughs. *Alternative Healing: The Complete A to Z Guide to Over 160 Alternative Therapies.* La Mesa, California: Halcyon Publishing, 1993.

Kleiner, Carolyn, "Mind-body Fitness: Yoga Booms in Popularity," *U. S. News & World Report*, May 13, 2002.

Lao Tzu. *Tao Te Ching.* Translated by D.C. Lau. New York: Viking Press, 1985.

Last Acts. *Means to a Better End: A Report on Dying in America Today.* Washington, D.C.: Last Acts, November 18, 2002

Levine, Steven. *Who Dies? An Investigation Of Conscious Living And Conscious Dying.* New York: Doubleday, 1982.

Lown, Bernard. *The Lost Art of Healing.* New York: Ballantine Books, 1999.

McCloud, John, "A Kinder, Gentler Death," *Time*, September 18, 2000.

National Center for Complementary and Alternative Medicine. U.S. Department of Health & Human Services. *Five Year Strategic Plan 2001–2005.* NIH Publication No. 01–5001. Silver Springs, Maryland: National Institutes of Health, September 25, 2000.

National Center for Complementary and Alternative Medicine. U.S. Department of Health and Human Services. *General Information.* Silver Springs, Maryland: National Institutes of Health, March 1997.

National Center for Complementary and Alternative Medicine. U.S. Department of Health and Human Services. *Alternative Medicine: expanding medical horizons.* Silver Springs, Maryland: National Institutes of Health, 1993.

National Sleep Foundation. *2005 Sleep in America Poll.* Washington, D.C.: National Sleep Foundation, March 29, 2005.

Pascal, Blaise. *Pensees.* Translated by A.J. Krailsheimer. New York: Penguin Classics, 1995.

Pert, Candace. *Molecules of Emotion: Why You Feel the Way You Feel.* New York: Scribner, 1997.

Plato (427–347 B.C.). Plato Complete Works. Edited by John M. Cooper and D.S. Hutchinson. Indianapolis, Indiana: Hackett Publishing Company, 1997.

Rinpoche, Sogyal. *The Tibetan Book Of Living And Dying.* San Francisco: HarperCollins, 1994.

Rose, Jeanne. *The Aromatherapy Book.* Berkeley, California: North Atlantic Books, 1992.

Rossbach, Sarah. *Interior Design With Feng Shui.* New York: Penguin Group, 2000.

Stapleton, Stephanie. "Medicine's Chasm: the wide gulf between conventional and alternative approaches," *American Medical News,* June 3, 2002.

Thurber, James (1894–1961), quotation attributed to an article in *New York Post,* February 29, 1960.

Tierra, Michael. *The Way of Herbs.* Santa Cruz, California: Unity Press, 1980.

Tierra, Lesley. *The Herbs of Life.* Freedom, California: Crossing Press, 1992.

Weil, Andrew, M.D. *Health and Healing.* Boston: Houghton Mifflin, 1983.

INDEX

Please note: *Page numbers in italics indicate illustrations.*

AIDS-related illnesses, 140
alternative medicine. *See also*
    providers, alternative
    medicine; remedies,
    alternative medicine
    about, 9–10, 21, 26, 94
    accessibility of, 10–11
    attitudes toward, 10, 49
    categories of, 92
    and chronic care health, 35, 36
    and condition of patients/
        consumers, 57
    confusion about, 31
    and costs, 93–94
    definition of, 25–26
    and emergency/non-emergency
        situations, 32–34
    and environment, healing,
        20–21
    framework/formula for using, 18
    and healing process, 21, 22
    and imbalance issues, 20, 32, 33
    and insurance benefits, health,
        34–35
    and organizations, 225–35
    and prevention of ill health,
        35, 36
    professional associations, 196,
        225–35
    and resources, Internet, 237–39
    summary, 222–23
    vs. conventional medicine,
        23–25, 26–27

American Academy of
    Environmental Medicine,
    124
appointments, medical, 47
aromatherapy, 195–99
attitudes of patients/consumers, 10,
    49, 157–63
Aurelius, Marcus *Meditations*, 210
ayurveda practice, 133–34, 143–45

Bach, Edward, 148
beverages and food. *See* nutrition
    issues
body work
    about, 178–79
    cartoon, 177
    craniosacral therapy, 182–83
    Energy Healing, 185
    Feldenkrais method, 183
    institutions, 182, 183
    massage therapy, 180–81
    Medical Qigong therapy,
        184–85
    organizations, 179, 183
    and osteopathic medicine, 179,
        182
    polarity therapy, 184
    professional associations, 181
    and professional associations,
        184, 185
    reading material/bibliography,
        176, 181
    summary, 90, 176

Therapeutic Touch℠, 185
workbook, 245
breathwork, 118–20, 121

cartoons
    body work, 177
    feng sui, 126
    internal energy work, 137
    lifestyle issues, 96
    mind work, 152
    soul work, 188
Centers for Disease Control and
    Prevention (CDC), 98
chemical sensitivity (MCS),
    multiple, 122
chronic care health, 35, 36
Clarke, Hulda, A Cure for all
    Disease, 123
consumer advocacy groups, 229
conventional medicine
    about, 26
    and doctors, 27–30, 79–80, 88
    and emergency/non-emergency
        situations, 32–34
    and imbalance issues, 32
    and negativity, 28–30
    and pharmacology, 35, 36
    and surgeries, 32, 35, 36
    vs. alternative medicine, 23–25,
        26–27
costs for services
    and alternative medicine, 93–94
    and alternative medicine
        remedies, 75
    death and dying issues, 214
    and providers, alternative
        medicine, 39
    and psychotherapists, 60, 62, 63
    and spiritual teachers, 60
Cousins, Norman, 174
craniosacral therapy, 182–83
Cure for all Disease, A (Clarke), 123

dana/donations, 60
death and dying
    and advance health care
        directives, 215
    and afterlife, 213–14

and attachments to life, 207–8
beliefs about, 205, 207–8
and costs, 214
fear of, 208
healing process, and approaches
    to, 206–7, 210
and home environment, 214
and hospice centers, 216
and hospital environment, 214
illnesses, and approaches to,
    205–6
and insurance benefits, health,
    215–16
and legal documents, 214–15
and mystical views of life,
    209–10
and Near Death Experience
    (NDE), 210
organizations, 216, 217, 229
professional associations, 229
reading material/bibliography,
    215, 217
and rebirth, 209–10
and spiritual inner life, 211–12
summary, 217
and unconditional love, 210–11
diet. See nutrition issues
diseases. See illnesses
doctors
    and alternative medicine
        remedies, 79–80, 88
    and conventional medicine,
        27–30, 49, 79–80, 88
    and health of patients/
        consumers, 16–17
    and patients/consumers, 38
    and providers, alternative
        medicine, 49
    vs. healers, 27–28

Einstein, Albert, 220
emergency/non-emergency
    situations, 32–34
Energy Healing, 185
energy work, external. See
    environmental balance
energy work, internal. See internal
    energy work

environmental balance. *See also*
environmental issues
about, 127–28, 133–34, 135
feng sui, 126, 128–31
organizations, 133–34, 135
and psychic energy practices,
134
reading material/bibliography,
125
summary of, 89, 125
vastu shastra, 131–34
workbook, 242
environmental issues
American Academy of
Environmental Medicine,
124
and cleaning up personal
environment, 124
death and dying in home
emvironment, 214
and environment, healing,
20–21
environmental illness (EI),
122
Environmental Protection
Agency (EPA), 122
and hospitals, 214
and lifestyle assessment, 121–24,
124
external energy work. *See*
environmental balance
Eysenck, Hans, 67

family psychotherapists, 58
fees for services
and alternative medicine, 93–94
and alternative medicine
remedies, 75
death and dying issues, 214
and providers, alternative
medicine, 39
and psychotherapists, 60, 62, 63
and spiritual teachers, 60
Feldenkrais, Moshe, 183
feng sui cartoon, 126
flower essence therapy, 147–49
food and beverages. *See* nutrition
issues

Hahnemann, Samuel, 141
healers vs. doctors, 27–28
healing process
about, 20–21
and active role of patients/
consumers, 220
and alternative medicine, 21, 22
and alternative medicine
remedies, 79, 88
and approaches to death and
dying, 206–7, 210
definition of, 219
and environment, healing,
20–21
and explanations, 220
and healing crises, 79, 88
multi-faceted approach to,
20–22
and opportunities for change
and growth, 220
and patients/consumers, active
role of, 220
and psychotherapists, 53–54, 69
six step plan, 89–91, 92–93
health, definition of, 21
health care, 35–36
health care crises, 220
health insurance benefits, 34–35,
215–16
Healthnotes Online, 75
herbalists
about, 74, 87
and alternative medicine
remedies, 74, 87
and combinations of herbs, 75
and freshness of herbs, 75
and internal energy work, 140
and organically grown herbs, 75
and surgeries, 194–95
and travel kit, 85–86
workbook, 249
Hering's Law of Cure, 142
Hippocrates, 29
hospitals, 201–2, 214

illnesses
and active role of patients/
consumers, 220

AIDS-related illnesses, 140
comprehensive approach to,
    19–20
death and dying, and
    approaches to, 205–6
and Energy Healing, 185
environmental illness (EI), 122
and imbalance issues, 205, 206
multi-faceted approach to, 19,
    21
multiple chemical sensitivity
    (MCS), 122
and personal experiences
    of alternative medicine
    providers, 45
and prevention of ill health,
    35, 36
and psychotherapists, 53–54
Seasonal Affective Disorder
    (SAD), 148
Therapeutic Touch℠, 185
imbalance issues. See also soul work
and alternative medicine, 20,
    32, 33
and ayurveda practice, 144
and biochemical imbalance, 59
and conventional medicine, 32
and craniosacral therapy, 182
and Eastern herbs, 80
and health imbalances, 80
and illnesses, 205, 206
and insomnia, 120
major imbalances, 32
and Medical Qigong therapy,
    184
minor imbalances, 33
and naturopaths, 146
physical imbalance, 30
and physical space, 129, 130,
    132
and polarity therapy, 184
information about health issues, 47,
    74–75, 237–39
inner life, 189–92
insurance benefits, health, 34–35,
    215–16
internal energy work
    about, 138

and acupuncture treatments,
    139, 140
and ayurveda, 143–45
cartoon, 137
and Chinese medicine, 138–41
and comprehensive methods
    and techniques, 147–49
flower essence therapy, 147–49
and herbal medicines, 140
and homeopathy, 141–43
light therapy, 147, 148, 149
and naturopathy, 145–47
organizations, 133–34, 141, 143,
    145, 147, 149
and osteopathic medicine, 147
reading material/bibliography,
    136, 148–49
sound therapy, 147, 148, 149
summary of, 90, 136
and Tibetan medicine, 147
workbook, 243
Internet resources, 237–39
Is Your Health Care Killing You?
    (Badell), 46

Kellogg, John, 146

Lao Tzu, 12, 221
Lennon, John, 221
lifestyle assessment. See also
    nutrition issues
and breath, using the, 118–20,
    121
and breathwork, 118–20, 121
and cleaning up personal
    environment, 124
and environment issues, 121–24
and exercise, 112–14
and insomnia, 120
and progressive relaxation
    training (PRT), 117
and quiet time, 116–20
reading material/bibliography, 95
and sleep, 120–21
and stress, 115–16
and stress issues, 115–16
summary of, 89, 95
workbook, 241

lifestyle issues, 74, 96, 97–98,
  221–22
light therapy, 147, 148, 149

marriage and family
  psychotherapists, 58
massage therapy, 180–81
medical appointments, 47
Medical Qigong therapy, 184–85
medicine, short history of, 6
meditation, 60, 150, 151, 161–63,
  197–98
Meditations (Aurelius), 210
mind work
  and attitude, 157–63
  cartoon, 152
  and connections, emotional,
    171–74
  and guided imagery, 165–67
  and humor, 174
  and hypnosis, 163–65
  and immune-building
    personality characteristics,
    155–57
  and journal writing, 150, 160–61
  and love, expressions of, 157–59
  and meditation, 150, 161–63,
    197–98
  organizations, 160, 161, 163,
    165, 167, 171, 175
  and prayer, 173–74
  and psychotherapists, 159–60
  reading material/bibliography,
    150–51
  and regression therapy, 167–71
  summary of, 90, 150–51
  and support groups, 172–73
  and thoughts, effects of, 153–55
  workbook, 244
"Mozart Fffect," 148, 198
multiple chemical sensitivity
  (MCS), 122
music therapy, 198–99
mystical views of life, 209–10

National Center for
  Complementary and
  Alternative Medicine, 25, 92

National Institutes of Health
  (NIH), 25
Near Death Experience (NDE),
  210
nutrition issues
  and alcoholic beverages, 110
  and carbohydrates, 99, 105–7
  and fats, 99, 101–4
  and healthy diets, 98–101,
    109–10
  and labels, food, 110
  and organic food, 104–5
  and protein, 99–100
  and salt, table, 107–8
  and smoking, 110
  and supplements, nutritional,
    111–12
  vegetarianism, 98, 100, 101–4
  and water, drinking, 108–9
  and weightloss, 100

past life regression therapy, 168–71
patients/consumers
  alternative medicine providers,
    and active role of, 46–47, 50
  attitudes of, 10, 49, 157–63
  condition of, 57, 69, 77–78, 79,
    80–87
  consumer advocacy groups, 229
  and doctors, 38
  healing process, and active role
    of, 220
  health care crises, and active
    role of, 220
  illnesses, and active role of, 220
  medical appointments, and
    active role of, 47
  providers, and health of, 16–17
  and psychotherapists, 57, 64–65,
    68, 69
  and records/reports, 47
  and research about health
    issues, 47
  and service assessments, 47–48,
    50
  and treatments, 47
perfection issues, 221
polarity therapy, 184

practices, alternative medicine,
    17–18, 31, 92–93
practitioners. *See* providers,
    alternative medicine
*Professional Therapy Never Includes
    Sex*, 64
progressive relaxation training
    (PRT), 117
providers, alternative medicine
    and active role of patients/
        consumers, 46–47, 50
    and alternative concepts,
        45–46, 50
    and approaches to treatments,
        39, 42, 50
    choosing, 39, 49–51
    and communication issues,
        43–44, 47–48
    and costs for services, 39
    and doctors, 49
    and education, 42–43, 50
    and face to face assessments,
        43–44
    and fraud, 46
    and health of patients/
        consumers, 16–17
    illnesses, and personal
        experiences of, 45
    and intentions, 44–45, 50
    and licenses, 41–42, 50
    and office/practice issues, 39
    and patients/consumers, 37–38
    and practice, longevity of, 43, 50
    and professionalism, 42, 48, 50,
        51, 225–36
    and profits, 46
    reading material/bibliography,
        50
    and referrals, 39–40, 50
    and resumes/CV's, 42
    and service issues, 47–48, 50
    and termination of service, 48,
        50
    and treatments, approach to, 39,
        42, 50
    workbook, 247
providers, conventional medicine.
    See doctors

psychiatrists, 58–59
psychic energy practices, 134
psychotherapists
    about, 58–59
    and associations, 70, 233–34
    and benefits of therapy, 65–66,
        69
    and bodymind concepts, 53–54,
        69
    choosing, 54–55, 69
    and compatibility with patients/
        consumers, 69
    and condition of patients/
        consumers, 57, 69
    and fees, 60, 62, 63
    and healing process, 53–54, 69
    and history of psychology, 61
    and home visits, 64
    and illnesses, 53–54
    and intentions, 62, 69
    and interpersonal issues, 63, 69
    and licenses, 59–60, 61, 69
    marriage and family
        psychotherapists, 58
    and memberships, professional,
        69
    and misconduct, professional,
        65, 66
    negative aspects of
        psychotherapy, 67–68
    and organizations, 233–34
    and partnerships with patients/
        consumers, 68
    past life regression therapy,
        168–71
    and personal issues, 63
    positive aspects of
        psychotherapy, 68
    and professionalism, 62, 65,
        66, 69
    and profits, 61
    psychiatrists, 58–59
    and referrals, 62
    and rights of patients/
        consumers, 64–65
    and techniques, 57
    and termination of therapy,
        65–66, 69

and tests, psychological, 59
and theoretical approaches,
56–57
and training, professional, 60,
61–62, 69
and transpersonal
psychotherapy, 56–57
vs. self directed personal growth,
68
and wellness model, 63
workbook, 248

Quarles, Francis, 5

records/reports, 47
regression therapy, 167–71
remedies, alternative medicine. *See
also* alternative medicine
about, 71–72
adverse reactions to, 79, 88
breaks from using, 78, 88
choosing, 72–74
and cold/hot packs, 85–86
and combinations of herbs, 75
and condition of patients/
consumers, 77–78, 79, 80–87
confusion about, 31
and costs, 75
directions for use of, 76–77, 87
and doctors, 79–80, 88
and Eastern remedies, 84–85
and expiration dates, 76
and freshness of herbs, 75
and harmful effects, 76
and healing crises, 79, 88
and herbalists, 74, 87
and herbal travel kit, 85–86
and homeopathic remedies, 81
and lifestyle issues, 74
and organically grown herbs, 75
and organizations, 88, 230–31
processing and standardization
of, 76
professional organizations,
230–31
reading material/bibliography,
87
and research, 74–75, 87

and teas, medicinal, 85
termination of use of, 79, 88
and Western remedies, 81–84
research about health issues, 47,
74–75
rest and relaxation
and breath, using the, 118–20,
121
and insomnia, 120
and progressive relaxation
training (PRT), 117
and quiet time, 116–20
and sleep, 120–21
and stress, 115–16

Seasonal Affective Disorder
(SAD), 148
service issues, patients/customers,
47–48, 50. *See also* fees for
services
sleep issues, 120–21
smoking issues, 110
soul work
about, 189–90
cartoon, 188
and prevention, 190–91
and professional associations,
191–92
and protection from influences,
190–91
purpose and meaning to life,
191–92
reading material/bibliography,
186–87, 191–92
summary, 90, 186–87
workbook, 246
and yoga practices, 190
sound therapy, 147, 148, 149
space, balancing individual. *See*
environmental balance
spiritual teachers, 60
Stone, Randolph, 184
stress issues, 115–16
supplements, nutritional, 111–12
surgeries
and alternative medicine, 32,
35, 36, 193–94
and anesthesiologists, 193, 194

and aromatherapy, 195–99
and conventional medicine, 32,
    35, 36
and emotional support, 200–201
herbs and supplements, 194–95
and hospitals, 201–2
and meditation, 151, 197–98
positive affirmations and
    statements, 199–200
reading material/bibliography,
    202–3
summary, 202–3
and surgeon, medical, 193–94

Tao Te Ching (Lao Tzu), 221
teachers, spiritual, 60, 158, 163,
    189, 190
Therapeutic Touch℠, 185
therapies. *See also* psychotherapists
    acupuncture treatments, 139,
        140
    aromatherapy, 195–96
    craniosacral therapy, 182–83
    Energy Healing, 185
    Feldenkrais method, 183
    flower essence therapy, 147–49
    massage therapy, 180–81
    Medical Qigong therapy,
        184–85
    music therapy, 198–99
    and organizations, 231–32, 233,
        234

past life regression therapy,
    168–71
polarity therapy, 184
professional associations,
    231–32, 233, 234
progressive relaxation training
    (PRT), 117
and psychiatrists, 58–59
regression therapy, 167–71
Therapeutic Touch℠, 185
Thurber, James, 174
treatments
    acupuncture treatments, 139,
        140
    and alternative medicine
        providers's approaches to, 39,
        42, 50
    and patients/consumers, 47
*12 Ways to Survive Our Fractured
    Health Care System* (Badell),
    46

Upledger, John, 182
U.S. Department of Agriculture,
    104, 106

vegetarianism, 98, 101–4

women's issues, 30

yoga practices, 190